THE MAN'S GUIDE TO GOOD HEALTH

THE MAN'S GUIDE TO GOOD HEALTH

Allen B. Weisse, M.D.

and the Editors of
Consumer Reports Books

CONSUMER REPORTS BOOKS
A Division of Consumers Union
Yonkers, New York

Library of Congress Cataloging-in-Publication Data
Weisse, Allen B.
    The man's guide to good health / Allen B. Weisse and the editors of Consumer Reports Books.
    p. cm.
    Includes index.
    ISBN 0-89043-303-8
    1. Men—Health and hygiene.   I. Consumer Reports Books.
    II. Title.
    RA777.8.W43   1991
    613'.0423—dc20   91-18886
                                                                 CIP

Design by GDS / Jeffrey L. Ward
Drawings by Robert McBride and John Karapelou
First printing, October 1991
Manufactured in the United States of America

This book is dedicated to
the three Charleses and
the one Clifford

Contents

Acknowledgments

A number of colleagues, many from the faculty of the New Jersey Medical School, have been kind enough to review the various chapters of this book as they neared completion. Special thanks to: Richard J. Francis, M.D.; Rajendra Kapila, M.D.; Eugene R. Kelly, M.D.; Phoebe R. Krey, M.D.; William A. Layman, M.D.; Reynard J. McDonald, M.D.; Jennifer Michaels, M.D.; James Minard, Ph.D.; Lillian F. Pliner, M.D.; Timothy J. Regan, M.D.; Robert A. Schwartz, M.D.; Joseph J. Seebode, M.D.; and Laura Weisse, M.D. Thanks also to Marilyn Bruder and Mimi Weaver. This is to acknowledge with gratitude their helpful criticisms, corrections, and suggestions for improvements.

A note of thanks also to Tom Blum, Julie Henderson, and others at Consumer Reports Books who assisted in shaping the book into its final form.

Finally, there is the debt all of us in medicine owe to our patients, from whom we continue to learn as we persist in attempting to serve them both wisely and well.

THE MAN'S
GUIDE TO
GOOD HEALTH

Introduction

Life expectancy for both men and women in the United States has gradually been increasing over the last few decades. In this respect, however, men have always lagged behind women, who tend to outlive them by about seven years on the average. One reason may be genetic, but another can be found in the general unwillingness of many men to confront their health problems realistically. Making changes in one's daily habits and general life-style can be painful, and some men adopt a fatalistic attitude toward illness and disease that may not serve them well in the long run.

This book attempts to remedy this situation, especially for those men who want to learn good health habits that will last a lifetime. Women, too, will find the information here valuable for the men in their lives, whether fathers, husbands, brothers, sons, or lovers.

We begin with the male musculoskeletal system—bones, joints, and muscles. Strains, sprains, bursitis, and various kinds of arthritis are common problems men encounter throughout their lives. Lower back pain and its relation to possible disk disease is also a major problem for many men, as are gout and a condition known as ankylosing spondylitis. Sports injuries are frequent among active men. All of these skeletal and muscular ailments are covered in chapter 1.

Coronary heart disease remains the number-one killer of American men. High blood pressure, by itself or in combination with heart disease, is no less important. In addition to these major threats, men are subject to valvular heart disease, diseases of the heart muscle (cardiomyopathies), and other rarer forms of heart problems. Details of diagnosis and current treatments are covered in chapter 2.

The techniques used to evaluate the heart patient are confusing to many, so this chapter explains the often difficult and technical diagnostic methods as clearly as possible. The variety of available medications used in cardiovascular disease is also bewildering—from simple aspirin to drugs that profoundly affect the strength of the heart's contractions, alter blood clotting mechanisms, and make changes in the production and distribution of fatty substances in the arteries. These potent and complicated drugs are explored in depth in this chapter, as are invasive procedures such as coronary bypass surgery and balloon angioplasty. Most important, the individual can learn how he can ensure that his heart remains healthy right up to old age.

After cardiovascular disease, no other type of illness poses a greater threat to American men than cancer. Cancer—its causes, types, warning signs, treatments—is discussed in chapter 3. Lung, colon, and prostate cancer are of special interest to men, but other rarer forms of cancer are also explored.

Disorders of the urinary tract are among the most common and disabling of male illnesses, especially with advancing age. These often chronic problems include prostatic enlargement, urinary retention, and susceptibility to prostatitis. Kidney stones can occur at any age, and they usually appear first in younger men. These and other maladies of the genitourinary system are covered in chapter 4.

The male sexual organs are closely related to the urinary tract. Chapter 5 covers many of the common disorders affecting these organs, including ejaculatory problems, infertility, and impotence. Since contraception is of paramount concern to both men and women, each available method of birth control, including vasectomy, is explored.

Sexually transmitted diseases remain a threat to all sexually active men, despite the ready availability of antibiotics. This is especially important because diseases such as syphilis and gonorrhea appear to be on the rise in certain segments of society. Other forms of venereal disease, such as genital herpes and chlamydia, are also more common. Hepatitis, not previously thought of as an STD, poses an even greater threat to long-term health and survival, exceeded only by the risk of AIDS. These diseases are fully discussed in chapter 5.

Mental and emotional illness represents a major cause of chronic disability for many men. The so-called mid-life crisis, in addition to the lifelong threats of acute anxiety, severe phobias, and mood disorders such as mania and depression, are covered in chapter 6. Sleep disorders can also cause a great deal of mental distress; information on sleep disturbances and what to do about them is found here.

Alcohol and drug abuse are now recognized as underlying causes of many mental problems and are covered in this chapter. Various types of psychotherapy and psychotropic drugs are also discussed.

Skin problems affect men of all ages—from minor irritations to acute inflammations and rashes. Among younger men, acne represents a major problem that can have debilitating physical and emotional consequences. Chapter 7 explores all of these skin ailments, including psoriasis and the various allergic reactions that first show up on the skin.

Excessive exposure to the sun has given rise to an alarming increase in skin cancer in the United States. The types of cancerous lesions and their prompt recognition and treatment are a major component of this chapter. Concerns about hair loss, a fact of life for most men as they age, are also discussed. For example, what are the current medical and surgical approaches to baldness? Are they any better than the nonmedical solutions offered by the cosmetic industry?

Elderly men can suffer major disruption in what are considered routine bodily functions: blockage of the urinary passage, a loss of bowel and bladder control, the failure of sight and hearing. But much has been learned about various practical, effective approaches to relieve and manage these aspects of aging. Chapter 8 discusses all the ways in which men can cope successfully with the physical changes that come with the years, and how new drugs and other physical therapies can help alleviate many of the disturbing symptoms experienced at this time of life.

Although they are inevitable, the challenges of aging are not necessarily all negative. This section can help a man to recognize the normal changes that occur as his mind and body grow older, and also outlines the personal measures necessary to prevent or reasonably forestall illness and disability in the later years.

Whatever the wonders of modern medicine, men cannot use them to advantage unless they understand how to deal effectively with the current health-care system. First, a man has to know how to choose the right physician for his needs. In what kind of setting does he wish to receive care: a solo practice, a small specialized group practice, or perhaps a large Health Maintenance Organization?

He must consider how he wants to pay for his medical treatment, not only for himself, but perhaps for his family as well. To do this effectively, he must get involved with the complexities of health insurance. At one time or another he may have other medical considerations. What are the steps to take before deciding upon major surgery? What can he expect once he is admitted to a hospital? What are his rights as a patient? The final chapter of this book answers all these important questions.

More than anything else, the intent of this book is to emphasize the importance to men of taking some of the responsibility for their own long-term physical and mental well-being. This commitment to good health requires that a man take an active (if not excessive) interest in his own health, that he make the necessary changes in his life-style that will foster good health habits, and that he cultivate a good working relationship with his personal physician and, if necessary, with other health professionals.

He will find that the results are usually worth the effort—namely, a long, productive, and enjoyable life.

1

Your Bones and Muscles and How They Work

THE SKELETAL SYSTEM

Our bony structures are the scaffold upon which the rest of the body is supported (see Figure 1.1). Sitting on the pelvis below, and supporting the skull above, it is the spine that allows for our upright posture. The spine consists of 33 separate bones (the vertebral column) divided into five major sections: the seven cervical vertebrae of the neck; the 12 thoracic vertebrae of the chest region; the five lumbar vertebrae, just behind the abdominal cavity; and the five sacral vertebrae, at the lowest point, to which are connected several small bones collectively called the coccyx (see Figure 1.2).

Because lower back problems are so common in men, it is important for you to understand the structure of the spine, especially the lumbar region, where many of these problems first occur. Other than in the sacrum (the lowest section of the spine), the vertebrae in the lumbar area are slightly movable in relation to one another, both above and below. This enables you to walk normally, maintain balance, bend, twist, and perform normal lifting. This mobility is made possible by the pres-

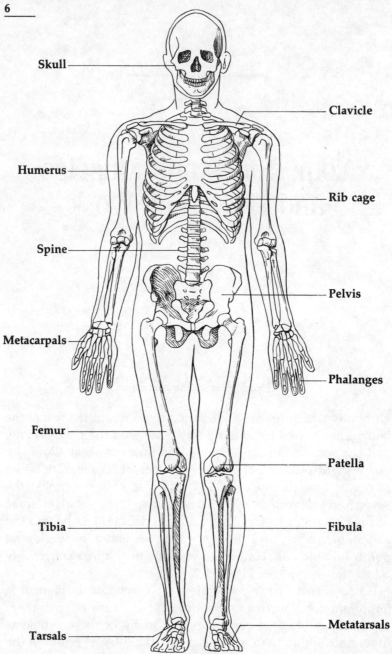

Skull

Clavicle

Humerus

Rib cage

Spine

Pelvis

Metacarpals

Phalanges

Femur

Patella

Tibia

Fibula

Tarsals

Metatarsals

Figure 1.1   The human skeleton

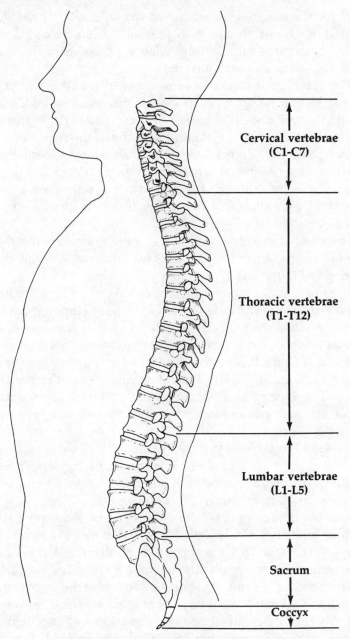

Figure 1.2 The vertebral column (lateral view)

ence between vertebrae of intervertebral disks. These disks consist of a hard, fibrous outer portion, within which is a soft, elastic gelatinous core. Besides allowing mobility of the spine, they also serve as shock absorbers.

The spinal cord runs in a canal formed by extensions of the vertebrae that rise from each side of the vertebral bodies and meet in the midline of the back. We can feel these ridges through the skin if we move our hand up and down the back along the spinal column. Nerve fibers, which account for both motor power and sensation, emerge from the spinal cord and pass in close proximity to the disks. If a disk protrudes onto a nerve root, both sensation and the ability to move specific muscles can be affected (see Figure 1.3).

The ribs begin at the back of the spine to encircle the chest, the upper ones inserting into the breastbone or sternum in the front (see Figure 1.1).

The other major areas of the skeletal system where problems often arise are in the long bones of the body, especially where they connect at the joints to provide freedom of movement. The typical movable joint is made up of two interconnecting bones, the ends of which are coated with a strong, resilient, pearly white cartilage. Powerful ligaments often hold the bones in place. This type of joint is surrounded by a thick capsule made up of the tendons of muscles that insert above and below into the long bones.

To keep the skeletal system operating well, the structure of the bones themselves must be maintained by ingesting normal amounts of calcium and other minerals and protein. Fortunately for most men, problems in this area are rare.

Another requirement is to maintain smooth movement at the various joints or articulations. This is aided by the normal bone molding that takes place with growth, so that the shapes of two interconnecting bones usually fit well with one another, and by the presence of the smooth cartilage surfaces at the points where bone surfaces meet. Most important to proper joint function is the presence of **synovial spaces**. These thin tissues or membranes contain a small amount of lubricating fluid to permit smooth and painless motion.

It is essential that the muscle of your extremities and spine remain in good tone because they support the joints and permit

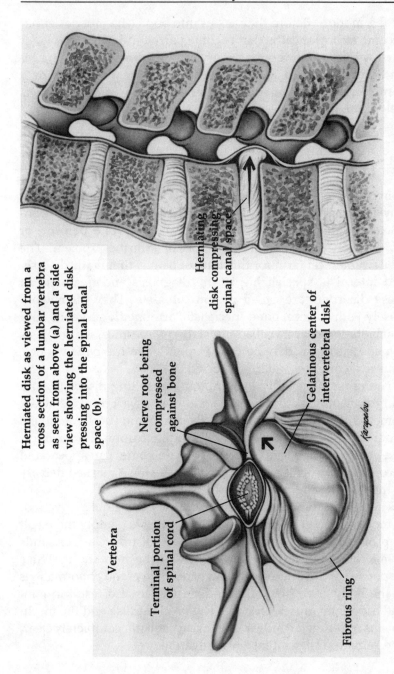

Herniated disk as viewed from a cross section of a lumbar vertebra as seen from above (a) and a side view showing the herniated disk pressing into the spinal canal space (b).

Herniating disk compressing spinal canal space

Figure 1.3B   Herniated disk (side view)

Vertebra

Nerve root being compressed against bone

Gelatinous center of intervertebral disk

Terminal portion of spinal cord

Fibrous ring

Figure 1.3A   Herniated disk (top view)

strong motion. Before they insert into bone, the muscles either become strong sheaths that become part of the joint capsule, or narrow into tough tendons. Tiny sacs or **bursae** containing lubricating fluid help reduce friction where tendons pass over bony surfaces during motion. Inflammation of these sacs is called **bursitis**.

DISORDERS OF THE MUSCULOSKELETAL SYSTEM

Pain in the joints, back, or muscles is one of the most frequent physical complaints of Americans. A national health survey conducted in 1987 estimated that approximately 14.6 percent, or 34.7 million people, had some sort of arthritic problem. The modern medical term for this type of pain is **rheumatic** disease, and internists specializing in the diagnosis and treatment of these disorders are called **rheumatologists**. They often work closely with surgical bone specialists, **orthopedic surgeons**, and rehabilitation doctors called **physiatrists**. At times, neurologists or neurosurgeons may be called upon when the patient's nervous system is secondarily affected.

The range of severity in symptoms, resulting disability, and long-term outlook for these conditions, as a group, is wide. Some aches and pains are relatively minor and transient; others progress slowly and only gradually impinge upon one's comfort and ability to cope; still others, fortunately rare, can appear and become severe with alarming speed, causing a marked debility of life-threatening proportions.

The causes of these arthritic diseases are similarly varied. Some may be degenerative in nature—that is, simply the result of prolonged wear and tear. Others result from various kinds of microbial infection or alterations in the immune system's response. Acute trauma can lead to disability, and abnormalities in the body chemistry of an individual can also result in joint and especially muscle disease. The precise cause and the mechanisms of certain arthritic problems are still not completely clear, and remain under intense investigation.

COMMON JOINT DISORDERS IN MEN: ARTHRITIS AND BURSITIS

Perhaps the last vestige of Latin in a modern doctor's training is his forced memorizaton of the four cardinal signs of inflammation: *dolor* (pain), *rubor* (redness), *tumor* (swelling), and *calor* (heat). If you have any of these symptoms in one of your joints, you don't need a medical degree to realize that you probably have some sort of an arthritic problem. The job for your physician is to locate the precise point of the problem, the particular abnormality, the cause of the problem, and finally, the best treatment. He or she will question you, examine you, and most often make an educated guess as to the severity of your condition and then recommend minor measures that will alleviate it. However, at times other means of diagnosis are called for.

X-ray examination of the skeletal system remains an invaluable ally to the doctor in determining whether you have arthritis or a related condition. Frequently, simple X rays of the body parts involved will reveal the abnormality causing the complaint. At other times, more sophisticated radiological techniques may be required; **computed tomography** (CT scanning) and **magnetic resonance imaging** (MRI) are currently producing spectacular pictures of these and other parts of the anatomy.

Occasionally, small amounts of radioactive substances will be injected intravenously and their subsequent concentration in various parts of the skeletal system observed by scanning the body. "Hot spots," those areas that pick up more of this material than do normal bones or joints, can indicate the presence of inflammation. **Arthrograms** have also been helpful in the past. These are obtained by injecting some radiopaque material (substances through which X rays cannot pass) within a joint and then taking X-ray pictures. For studies of the spinal canal, oftentimes for disk disease, **myelograms** are obtained in a similar way, with injection of the material into the spinal canal. To a large extent, however, these tests are being replaced by the noninvasive CT and MRI studies.

Often the cause of an inflamed joint or bursa is not clear. If excess fluid is present, the rheumatologist may insert a needle into a swollen joint and extract some of the fluid. Not only does this help to relieve the discomfort but, by examining the fluid under the microscope, culturing it, and doing cell counts and certain other chemical tests, the rheumatologist can focus in on the problem with much greater precision.

It may also help to look directly into a joint with an **arthroscope**, an instrument that allows visualization of internal structures not seen as well by other types of examination. A biopsy of the synovial membrane surrounding a joint, or bone substance, can also provide important diagnostic information in selected instances. If the rheumatic problem arises in the muscle rather than in the bone or joint, a muscle biopsy can be performed under local anesthesia.

Degenerative Arthritis (Osteoarthritis)

This is, without doubt, the most common rheumatic disease—unfortunately we all "rust" with age. In more scientific terms, the cartilage at the ends of bones, especially the weight-bearing bones, becomes soft and worn away. It also becomes pitted and distorted through wear and tear. This condition is often accompanied by the formation of bony spurs at joint margins, and the synovial membrane that faciliates movement may become mildly inflamed. The knee, hip, and spine are particularly prone to the effects of long, hard use. Hands and feet may also be affected.

There is a good deal of variation in our susceptiblity to osteoarthritis, some of it probably genetic in nature. One factor that also may play a part is obesity. And certain stressful occupations may make particular individuals susceptible to osteoarthritis—the spine in coal miners, for example, or the shoulders of bus drivers. Any joint that has been previously damaged in some way may become the site of premature osteoarthritis. The aches and pains of osteoarthritis include persistent pain or occasional soreness and swelling in the joints. Fever accompanying joint pains is unusual and suggests another reason for the arthritis.

Treatment of Arthritis

Osteoarthritis is so common a disorder that many who have a mild case treat it at home without any special medical assistance. When symptoms are severe enough to warrant a visit to the doctor, X rays sometimes are used to confirm that it is osteoarthritis and not some other condition. The extent of the disease can also be ascertained in this way. Medication in some form is often necessary for relief of symptoms.

Pain-relieving drugs. Since almost all the conditions that come under the heading of arthritis are painful, the use of drugs to relieve pain and inflammation is common. Given the frequency of such complaints, it is no wonder that a flip of the television dial is likely to reveal yet another advertisement of some new remedy for the relief of back pain, arthritis, or some other musculoskeletal problem.

Aspirin remains an effective and inexpensive agent for the relief of many minor aches and pains; it can also lower body temperature when fever is present, and directly reduce inflammatory reactions.

Unfortunately, many people cannot tolerate aspirin; they experience upper abdominal discomfort and nausea when they take it. Aspirin can also cause small erosions in the lining of the stomach and occasionally result in significant blood loss. To overcome such difficulties, especially if aspirin needs to be used for a prolonged period, special preparations are available, such as buffered aspirin (Bufferin) or coated tablets (Ecotrin).

An alternative to aspirin is **acetaminophen**, a different kind of pain reliever. Available over-the-counter (Tylenol, Anacin), it is probably the most widely used analgesic on the market today. Although popular and effective for both pain relief and fevers, acetaminophen has no significant anti-inflammatory action (as compared to aspirin), and so is less useful in the treatment of diseases such as bursitis and certain kinds of arthritis.

The introduction of **steroids** or cortisone-like drugs in the 1950s initially offered great promise for arthritis sufferers. But though potent as anti-inflammatory agents, the steroids were soon found to have many serious side effects, especially with long-term use:

- They interfere with the body's defense against infections.
- They cause fluid retention, serious weight gain, and disruptions of the normal balance of sodium and potassium.
- They cause duodenal ulcers.

• They interfere with the control of glucose in known diabetics, and precipitate the disease in others.
• They cause muscle weakness and bone destruction.
• In rare instances, they cause or contribute to serious mental disturbances.

Although some of the newer steroid preparations are tailored to address a patient's specific needs, most of these dangerous side effects have never been eliminated. Therefore, these drugs are prescribed for only a limited number of life-threatening conditions and for the shortest length of time and the lowest effective dose schedule possible.

Because local injection of cortisone preparations (as opposed to taking them orally) does not ordinarily affect the body as a whole, physicians use such injections for various inflammatory conditions, especially tendinitis.

Nonsteroidal anti-inflammatory drugs (NSAIDs) entered the drug market in the 1970s to fill the gap between the older analgesics such as aspirin and the often too-potent steroid preparations. These NSAIDs include **indomethacin** (Indocin), **ibuprofen** (Motrin, Advil, Nuprin, Mediprin), **naproxen** (Naprosyn), **sulindac** (Clinoril), **piroxicam** (Feldene), and **diclofenac** (Voltaren), among others. Although they are potent against pain and inflammation, these drugs do have some side effects that are often not fully explained to patients receiving them.

One major problem is that such drugs often provoke upper gastrointestinal symptoms similar to those caused by aspirin. Also, like aspirin, they can cause gastrointestinal bleeding. They also can have a damaging effect upon the kidneys, often in patients previously unaware of any kidney problem. Fortunately, the kidney malfunction is usually reversible when the offending drug is stopped.

Because of the potentially serious side effects of NSAIDs, many physicians are concerned now that they have become available as over-the-counter drugs. Although the recommended dosage on these package inserts is much lower than that ordinarily prescribed by physicians, overuse of these agents is a real possibility, especially since many people are now taking

NSAIDs as the first drug for relief of musculoskeletal pain. Remember, the older pain relievers are still effective for most conditions. They are also cheaper, and their various side effects are much better understood and recognized. NSAIDs, even in the smaller dosages recommended in over-the-counter preparations, are potent drugs, and this potency should be respected. Never exceed the recommended period of time you take the drug before consulting a physician. If you encounter any new sensation, pain, or discomfort, discontinue use and seek medical advice for the problem.

Because of the potential dangers of steroids, the drug **phenylbutazone** (Butazolidin) seemed a good alternative when it was introduced 25 to 30 years ago. Unfortunately, in some patients, it was found to cause anemia and drops in the white blood cell count due to bone marrow depression. It is rarely used today. Question your doctor carefully if he or she prescribes this drug for you.

Antibiotics have no role in the treatment of arthritic disease unless the basis for the disease is a bacterial infection. For special rheumatic problems affecting the body as a whole (systemic diseases) and not just limited to the bones or joints, steroids may be used with care. Other agents such as **gold, azathioprine, chloroquine, methotrexate, colchicine**, and **allopurinol** are also reserved for these very specific problems.

Other forms of treatment. Though the range of drugs now available for relief of pain and inflammation is impressive, physical therapy, rest, and, at times, exercise are often essential components in the treatment of arthritis and related conditions. Heat, electrical stimulation, and whirlpool treatments can be used alone or in combination with drug therapy in the management of these conditions. Occasionally the use of a cane may help reduce the weight load on the joints of the lower extremities. Splints may also be part of the treatment.

Surgical treatment is indicated only rarely, and only for very severe and deforming disease, usually involving the knees or hips. Total replacement of knee or hip joints is among the most important milestones of orthopedic surgery during the last two decades, and has literally given some arthritis sufferers new leases on a useful life.

Gout

Except for occasional occurrences among postmenopausal women, gout is predominantly a disease of adult men. Gout usually conjures up visions of an overweight, crotchety individual nursing a hot and exquisitely tender joint, usually at the base of a big toe. The real problem, however, is more complicated, and stems from an irregularity in the way some persons handle substances called purines and their metabolic product, uric acid.

Gout is caused by one of two types of defect. Either there is an overproduction (5 to 10 percent of all cases) or an underexcretion (90 to 95 percent of cases) of urate in the urine. Both conditions fall under the heading of **primary gout**. When amounts of urate accumulate as a result of other conditions, the disease is called **secondary gout**. Among these other conditions are certain disorders of the blood, and kidney failure. Secondary gout may also follow administration of certain drugs prescribed for other conditions (see below). There is also a type of chronic lead poisoning that can result in one form of secondary gout. This is called **saturnine gout**, referring to its frequency among the ancient Romans, who drank wine from vessels made from alloys containing a high percentage of lead; the acid in the wine leached lead from these vessels, so that it was imbibed with the wine.

Symptoms and diagnosis. Over 50 percent of those who come down with gout experience sudden pain at the base of a big toe as the first symptom. The pain is accompanied by warmth, redness, and swelling of the affected joint. In about 90 percent of gout sufferers, the big toe is eventually affected (a condition called **podagra**), although other joints may also be involved, usually those of the lower extremities (feet, instep, knee).

In an acute attack, urate crystals become deposited in the synovial space of a joint. These crystals incite an inflammatory reaction in which white blood cells play an important role. The pain of these attacks is usually so severe as to suggest some kind of acute infection. The attack often occurs unexpectedly in the middle of the night and may be triggered by trauma, heavy drinking, other drugs (especially diuretics), or even other illnesses.

A positive diagnosis of gout requires a finding of urate crystals by microscopic examination of the joint fluid. Your doctor can do this about 90 percent of the time. When this is unsuccessful for one reason or another, suspicion of gout can be strengthened by the character of the attack, the joint involved, and the level of uric acid in the blood. A family history of gout also helps to confirm the diagnosis. Finally, a patient's dramatic response to one of the traditional treatments for gout, **colchicine**, is strong evidence that gout is the culprit.

The level of uric acid in the blood is not always as helpful in diagnosis as one might presume. It can be normal during an acute attack and elevated at other times, even in arthritic diseases that are not gouty in nature. Elevated uric acid levels are also present in about 5 percent of Americans *without* gout. Such elevations may be without discernible cause or may result from kidney failure or drugs commonly used for the treatment of high blood pressure or fluid retention: **thiazides** (Diuril and Hydrodiuril) and **furosemide** (Lasix).

In well-established gout, X rays taken of the affected joint may show typical "punched out" lesions of the bone as well as other changes within the affected joint.

Once the diagnosis of primary gout is made, your doctor can determine by urine and blood tests whether it is because of overproduction or underexcretion of urate. This information may help in the future management of the problem and in the selection of drug therapy.

Complications. Besides the severe arthritis that may result from repeated flare-ups of gout in a joint, collections of urate crystals may form nodules under the skin (**tophi**) and in various parts of the body. Nodules usually mean that treatment for the gout has been inadequate over a long period of time. Further complications can occur if urate deposits in the kidney injure this organ. The incidence of uric acid stones is also seven or eight times higher in gout sufferers than in those with normal levels of uric acid in the blood. (About 10 to 20 percent of gout patients will ultimately experience the latter complication.)

High blood pressure and coronary heart disease also may be higher among those with gout, especially in those who are overweight.

Treatment. Treatment of gout is divided into several phases:

relief of the acute attack; prevention of further acute attacks; and prevention or reversal of the effects of urate deposits in and around the joints, under the skin, or within the kidney.

An acute attack can often be terminated by colchicine given either intravenously or by mouth. An alternative is the use of NSAIDs, which are very effective in this situation. For the rare acute attacks of gout that do not subside despite such measures, short-term dosage of phenylbutazone or a cortisone medication may be the final option. These are rarely needed, however. Prevention of future attacks can be accomplished through regularly scheduled prophylactic use of colchicine.

Drugs to rid the body of excess uric acid by increasing excretion through the kidney (uricosuric agents) can prevent further attacks of gout, as well as reduce the likelihood of complications. Primary among these uricosuric agents are **probenecid** (Benemid) and **sulfinpyrazone** (Anturane). Interaction of these drugs with other drugs is common, so careful monitoring for side effects is important. Aspirin presents special problems for the gout sufferer. It will block the uricosuric action of both probenecid and sulfinpyrazone, and, taken by itself even in moderate doses (e.g., up to six tablets a day), will interfere with the excretion of uric acid, thereby raising blood levels and increasing the chances of acute attacks. It seems prudent, therefore, for those with gout to avoid the routine use of aspirin.

Gout presents other special dangers in the area of drug interactions. Because acute attacks are episodic, it is possible to forget to mention the condition to a doctor treating you for an altogether different ailment. It is therefore particuarly important with gout patients that before you take any prescription or over-the-counter medication, you know its effect on uric acid levels. Read the material supplied with the drug carefully, and when in doubt consult your doctor.

Besides using uricosurics to help the kidneys get rid of uric acid, another option is to block the metabolic steps that lead to uric acid production. **Allopurinol** (Zyloprim) is effective in doing this. The choice for chronic therapy must often be made between the uriocosuric agents and allopurinol. Both types of drug do often interact with other medications, and the frequency of side effects is about the same with each type. When side effects do occur, however, they tend to be somewhat more severe with allopurinol, and for this reason some rheumatologists may prefer to start the therapy with uricosurics. On the other hand, allopurinol becomes the drug of choice for those in whom some kidney damage has already occurred, a condition that might be aggravated by suddenly increased uric acid loads to the kidney following the use of uricosurics.

What to do if you have gout. At one time, the gouty patient was usually portrayed as a portly, self-indulgent glutton, the victim of his own excesses. Actually the relationship of obesity to gout is not clear, although gout sufferers have fewer attacks when they lose weight. As for types of food that may contribute to gout, very few foods in the modern American diet are high in purines, the substances that are ultimately converted to uric acid; with the exception of restricting liver and other organ foods, no major dietary prohibitions are likely to be imposed on a gout patient. However, alcohol decreases urate excretion and may precipitate acute attacks, so restriction of alcohol intake is advised. Good fluid intake is helpful in maintaining adequate hydration and in avoiding overconcentration of the urine. It is especially important in preventing urinary tract stones when probenecid is prescribed.

Perhaps the most important contribution of the patient toward his own welfare is to acknowledge that he has a lifelong, incurable problem that can only be managed successfully with his continued understanding and cooperation. While there is no cure for gout, the disease can be properly managed, and it need not diminish the quality of life or interfere with the rewards of an active and productive life-style.

Rheumatoid Arthritis

Although classified among diseases of the joints, rheumatoid arthritis is actually a systemic disease that involves many parts of the body. Problems in the joints represent only the most impressive and obvious manifestations of the disorder. Though the disease is three times more common in women than in men, it may be present in as many as one person per every hundred of the population, and so is by no means a rare disease among men.

Symptoms. The onset and severity of rheumatoid arthritis can be highly variable. In some instances the condition may run its course over a period of months; in others it may involve decades of pain and disability. The cause of the disease is not known. The joints most commonly involved—usually on both sides of the body—are those of the hands, wrists, and feet. Gradual swelling, redness, and tenderness in these joints usually precipitate a visit to the doctor's office. Morning stiffness, an inability to get moving without discomfort and aching, is typical of rheumatoid arthritis; the extent of morning stiffness is often an indication of the overall severity of the disease.

Because rheumatoid arthritis involves the entire body, generalized symptoms such as simply feeling ill (malaise) and fatigue are part of the syndrome. In about 20 percent of those afflicted, nodules form under the skin, often at the elbows. The inflammatory process can also involve the pericardium, the sac around the heart, produce lung changes, and involve the eyes and nervous system. If untreated or inadequately treated, rheumatoid arthritis can progress to severe destruction of the joints, leading ultimately to confinement to bed or a wheelchair, as well as to a host of other problems over time. Fortunately, such severe complications occur in only 10 percent of all those who have the disease.

Treatment. The drug treatment plan for rheumatoid arthritis is frequently set up as a pyramid, with the first line of conservative therapy at the base, and an upward progression to more potent therapy as the patient encounters a more severe form of the disease. In milder cases, drugs such as aspirin and NSAIDs may suffice. For those who do not respond to such therapy, steroids, gold preparations, and antimalarial drugs (such as **chloroquine**) may be employed. A derivative of penicillin called **penicillamine** or drugs affecting the immune system or specific metabolic pathways produce some benefit in some patients. Azathioprine (Imuran) and methotrexate are in the latter category.

It is essential that physical therapy accompany every level of drug therapy. Rest and exercise including hydrotherapy (swimming and whirlpool baths) can help keep the individual functioning. Orthopedic and rehabilitation doctors may order other kinds of treatment, including the use of splints, braces, and other devices. Finally, in the most severe cases, joint reconstruction by an orthopedic surgeon may become necessary.

Ankylosing Spondylitis (AS)

AS is now recognized as similar to an ancient disease that has been found in some Egyptian mummies and that may have been the prototype for modern AS. The disease is now placed at the head of a group of disorders called **spondylarthropathies** (spinal arthritis).

Unlike rheumatoid arthritis, with which it was once mistakenly confused, AS is predominantly a disease of men. It is an inheritable disease: A substance on the cell membrane called HLA-B27 is found in more than 95 percent of affected white males. The onset is usually between the late teen years and age thirty. The lower spine and expecially the sacroiliac joints (see Figure 1.2) are prominently affected, causing pain and morning stiffness. AS tends to involve joints that are composed mostly of cartilage, so it is the intervertebral disks and the joints between the ribs and the vertebrae that first become inflamed and later fuse and calcify.

Over a period of years the spine and rib cage become rigid, and motion is limited. Anti-inflammatory drugs and exercise are prescribed to prevent fusion of the joints. In more severe cases, drugs such as **asulfadine** or methotrexate may be given. With proper treatment, most men with AS can lead normal lives. Occasionally they must change their line of work, especially if lifting, bending, and prolonged standing are a required part of their employment.

Infectious Arthritis

A number of infectious agents (bacteria, viruses, and other microbes) may settle in one or more joints, causing sudden inflammation and potential destruction of cartilage and bone. Fortunately, prompt recognition and treatment can often lead to complete recovery.

One clue leading to a diagnosis of infectious arthritis is that usually only one joint is involved; for someone with no previous history of arthritis, a single joint suddenly swells and becomes tender and warm. A fever and a generalized feeling of illness may accompany the joint pain. The doctor, suspecting infection, will obtain a specimen of the fluid within the joint, using a needle and syringe. Observing a sample under the microscope and performing a white cell count, he or she can often confirm the bacterial infection, and appropriate antibiotic therapy can begin.

Infectious arthritis is caused by various bacteria, each with its own pathology:

Staphylococci. Infectious arthritis is often caused by this type of bacteria. Common residents of the skin, staph germs can enter a joint through penetrating cuts or other wounds. But most often, because of the rich blood supply to the joints of the body, staphylococci gain entrance to a joint through the bloodstream. This condition is treated with antibiotics.

Gonococci. For the sexually active, gonorrhea is the most common culprit in infectious arthritis, with joint involvement in one to five of every thousand men infected with gonorrhea. The knee seems to be a favorite joint for gonococcal arthritis to settle in, although **arthralgia** (pain without redness or swelling) in other joints is often present. About two-thirds of men with gonococcal arthritis will also have skin lesions, small papules, or blisters. It is important to recognize that the arthritis may occur without a painful urethral discharge, the most common clinical symptom of gonorrhea. In about 75 percent of men with gonococcal arthritis, the organism can be cultured from the urethra, even when it is difficult to culture it from the joint fluid itself. The condition is treated with antibiotics, usually given intravenously for maximal effect.

Reiter's syndrome. This disorder involves three organ systems. The symptoms include those of arthritis, urethritis, and conjunctivitis. It is almost entirely a disease of men and, like ankylosing spondylitis, is associated with the HLA-B27 gene locus.

Symptoms usually start two to three weeks following a nonbacterial genital infection or severe diarrhea. It begins as an inflammatory arthritis involving the ankles, knees, and feet, and it may be preceded by a painful urethral discharge (urethritis).

Irritation of the eyes (conjunctivitis) may be a part of the picture. A number of individuals with Reiter's syndrome will experience lower back pain similar to that of ankylosing spondylitis. NSAIDs are helpful, but in the 10 to 20 percent of those men with eye symptoms, instillation of steroids into the eye is necessary. Although related to prior infection, the infecting agent is not a bacterium, and so Reiter's is not relieved by the administration of antibiotics.

Lyme disease. The name of this form of arthritis derives from the Connecticut town where it was first characterized as a distinct disease, although the disease has probably existed throughout the world for some time now. A small spiral-shaped organism called a **spirochete** is transmitted to humans by the bite of a tick that previously fed on one of the common wildlife carriers of the spirochete, usually deer or mice.

The initial symptom, occurring between three and 30 days after a bite, is an expanding red lesion (often with a distinct, paler center) at the site of the wound, although this may be so mild as to go unnoticed. Pain, without redness or swelling, is frequently present early in the disease and, if left untreated, can progress into full-blown arthritis. The nervous system, eyes, and heart may become involved. It is important to recognize the disease early so that treatment with antibiotics can begin promptly.

The diagnosis of many infectious diseases involves isolation of the attacking organism from a visible lesion or from the bloodstream, but in Lyme disease this has rarely been successful. For this reason, increasing reliance has been placed on blood testing for the presence of antibodies to the spirochete causing the disease. Such testing is not as reliable as we'd like to see it; many false-negative results occur, especially early in the disease, when sufficient amounts of antibody may not yet be present. As Lyme disease continues to spread, efforts are being made to improve the laboratory diagnosis. Until this happens, your doctor has to rely on what information you provide, and on what your doctor observes of your symptoms.

Other causes of infectious arthritis. Tuberculosis, once a common disease, has long been recognized as a cause of infectious arthritis. With the declining incidence of TB in the United

States, this type of arthritis has become rare. TB again seems to be on the rise, however, especially in crowded urban centers, so we may be seeing more of its complications.

Rheumatic fever, which follows a certain type of streptococcal infection, can also cause arthritis. This type has also become relatively rare, although, again, recent isolated outbreaks of rheumatic fever in several parts of the country have given some cause for renewed concern.

The early pattern of symptoms of some forms of hepatitis can feature arthritic symptoms. Once inflammation of the liver becomes apparent, however, these symptoms are recognized as expressions of hepatitis rather than of one of the other forms of arthritis.

COLLAGEN VASCULAR DISEASES

A group of diseases known as collagen vascular diseases are somewhat related to rheumatoid arthritis and some other forms of arthritis. What distinguishes the collagen vascular diseases is that they often prominently affect the skin and certain vital organs, such as the heart, kidney, and lung. As a result, the complications of collagen disease may at times be life-threatening. All three major collagen vascular diseases are much less common, however, in men than in women.

Systemic Lupus Erythematosis

The name of this disease derives from the redness (*erythema*) over the cheeks of many patients that eventually develops into a pattern occasionally reminiscent of the facial markings of the wolf (*lupus*). Lupus is an autoimmune disease; antibodies, for reasons not fully understood, are produced in the body of the patient and then proceed to attack the patient's own tissues.

Although several organ systems may be involved, the severity of the disease can vary widely from patient to patient. Joint pain is frequently the first sign of the disease, along with the facial rash. The most common cardiac complication, occurring in as many as one-third of all lupus patients, is inflammation of the sac around the heart (pericarditis). The lung and its lining may become involved, as well as the brain. It is the kidney, however, that holds the key to the final outcome, with the extent of renal damage the best predictor of the patient's chances for survival.

Because of the inflammatory nature of the disease, nonsteroidal anti-inflammatory drugs (NSAIDs) are often the first line of defense. When these are ineffective, **hydroxychloraquine** (Plaquenil) is often used. When vital organs become involved, steroids, which interfere with the immune response, may be required. Other agents, such as **azathioprine** (Imuran) or **cyclophosphamide** (Cytoxan), may also play a role in more resistant cases.

One particular form of lupus, of special pertinence to men, is drug-induced lupus erythematosis. There are a number of drugs frequently used in men that can, on rare occasions, cause symptoms that in all clinical ways are similar to classic lupus.

The most common offender is **procainamide** (Pronestyl), an effective antiarrhythmic drug that has often been used to suppress potentially life-threatening irregularities of the heartbeat, especially in men with coronary heart disease. About half of those taking procainamide on a regular basis will eventually develop antinuclear antibodies, characteristic of lupus, in their bloodstreams. Fortunately, a much smaller number of these will develop a lupus syndrome. Although the condition is reversible upon withdrawal of the offending drug, the symptoms can be severe and require intense treatment.

Other drugs less frequently reported to cause a lupus syndrome include the sulfa drugs, penicillin, anticonvulsants (Dilantin), **isoniazid** (used to treat tuberculosis), the antihypertensive **alpha methyl dopa** (Aldomet), and a drug commonly used for the treatment of hyperthyroidism, **propylthiouracil**. At one time, **hydralazine** (Apresoline), a drug useful in the treatment of resistant hypertension and heart failure, developed a reputation for precipitating lupus symptoms when prescribed in relatively high doses. There is now a limitation on the prescribed dosage of this drug, and this complication has been virtually eliminated.

Scleroderma (Systemic Sclerosis)

Progressive systemic sclerosis is a disorder characterized by excessive buildup of fibrous connective tissue. In this condition, for some reason, the process that regulates the cells that make collagen, or fibrous connective tissue, goes out of control. Scleroderma is primarily a disease of the skin, but complaints commonly involve the joints (puffiness and pain), especially of the hands. One striking early symptom can be a bluish discoloration of the skin after exposure to cold (**Raynaud's phenomenon**). Later on, the skin becomes tight and thickened, giving the face a wizened appearance, especially around the nose and cheeks. The upper gastrointestinal tract is often involved, and there may be problems with swallowing or regurgitation of acidic contents from the stomach back into the esophagus, causing esophagitis. An X ray often reveals the typical widened appearance of the esophagus in such instances.

Scleroderma occurs most often between the ages of 30 and 60. Like lupus, the range of severity in scleroderma is wide. Treatment is directed to reducing the amount of fibrous tissue produced by the disease, along with physical therapy to provide relief of symptoms and to maintain as near normal function as possible.

Polymyositis and Dermatomyositis

Although the causes may be different, these two diseases are often linked together because of their frequent coexistence. The least common of the major collagen disorders, polymyositis, primarily involves inflammation of the muscles, while dermatomyositis prominently involves the skin, where symptoms may appear before, during, or after the onset of the muscle inflammation. In general, the outlook, following intense treatment with steroids, is quite good.

LOWER BACK PAIN

It is estimated that about 80 percent of Americans will, at one time or another, experience lower back pain. Lower back pain is one of the most common, expensive, and exasperating medical problems confronting American men. It is topped only by headaches, colds, and flu as a major cause of absence from work. The entire age spectrum, from young men to old, may be severely incapacitated by the symptoms of lower back pain.

Many of the arthritic conditions already discussed involve the back. Osteoporosis, a loss of structural bone support in the spinal column, is a common cause of such pain among older women. Degenerative arthritis (osteoarthritis) can result in similar symptoms and can occur simultaneously with osteoporosis. Several relatively rare diseases occur in the bones of the spinal column. Cancers can spread to these areas, causing bone destruction and pain, as can trauma to the back as a result of obvious accidents. Rarely, the cause of pain in the lower back will be an infection taking hold in that location.

All of these well-established causes of lower back pain must be considered as possibilities by your doctor. However, the overwhelming number of cases of lower back pain will fall into the category commonly labeled "lower back strain or sprain." (A strain is an overstretching of a muscle; a sprain involves some tearing of muscle or ligament fibers. Neither is identifiable by X-ray examination.) The area involved corresponds to that of the lumbosacral region (see Figure 1.2), and although the precise anatomic lesion may not be identified, the problem is generally agreed to be mechanical in nature.

In a much smaller number of individuals, one or more types of X-ray study will reveal that the problem is related to a demonstrable disease of one or more intervertebral disks and adjacent bony structures of the spine—popularly known as "slipped disk(s)". Let's look at two types of lower back pain, one unrelated to disk trouble, and the other caused by a herniated disk.

Lower Back Pain (Non-disk-Related)

Much of the pain that falls into this category can be and frequently is self-treated by the individual affected, especially if the problem is of short duration and responsive to the usual measures of rest and over-the-counter pain medications.

To rule out serious disk disease, the back-pain sufferer should ask himself the following questions:

- Has the pain lasted more than a week, despite attempts to treat it with bed rest and over-the-counter anti-inflammatory medications?
- Does the back pain seem to be related to a recent accident?
- Does the pain shoot down the back of the leg (sciatica)?
- Is there any loss of strength or sensation in the legs?
- Is there any loss of urinary or bowel control?
- Is fever a prominent symptom?

A "yes" to any one of the above questions may indicate that the problem involves more than just a simple back strain or sprain, and calls for physical examination by a doctor. If a severe strain or sprain seems the most likely cause, the doctor may order blood tests, which reveal evidence of muscle damage, but usually he or she will not order X rays. Unless the symptoms create a strong suspicion of bone pathology, experts discourage the use of expensive (and not altogether harmless) X-ray studies in those under the age of 50. Even in acute lower back pain accompanied by pain and tenderness along the nerve that runs down the back of the thigh, the likelihood of disk disease or other bone involvement is low.

Treatment. In view of the usually good outlook for those with acute lower back pain (no more than six weeks in duration), conservative treatment should be the rule. Strict bed rest is an important element of treatment. At one time, two weeks of bed rest were routinely prescribed. Recent controlled studies have shown, however, that one week or even less may be equally effective. The patient should use various types of over-the-counter pain-relieving analgesics, such as aspirin, ibuprofen, and acetaminophen. Hot or cold applications to the affected areas are also recommended. After recovery, the patient should take measures to prevent a recurrence—avoiding improper methods of lifting, pursuing possible weight reduction, and doing exercises to strengthen the muscles of the back and abdomen.

Chronic Lower Back Pain (Non-disk-Related)

After three months from the onset of lower back symptoms, only 5 percent of individuals will continue to complain of pain. Other sufferers who achieved initial relief will have had one or more recurrences of the original condition. Such persistent pain increases the likelihood of structural spine disease. At this point X-ray studies of the spine are usually recommended. These may include standard X rays of the spine in various views, computed tomography (CT scan), myelography, and magnetic resonance imaging (MRI). Computed tomography, especially with myelography, is generally the most reliable of these current methods. At this time the patient should probably consult a rheumatologist, neurologist, or surgical specialist in orthopedics or neurosurgery.

If all of this testing results in a diagnosis of a noncorrectable disease, your physician will recommend a continuance of conservative treatment, perhaps more intensive. Special exercises, despite some persistence of pain, are occasionally of great benefit.

Herniated Disk Disease

Disk herniation refers to a protrusion of the disk beyond its normal confines (see Figure 1.2). Although disk herniation has been found rather frequently in individuals with no symptoms of lower back pain or sciatica (20 percent in one study), when it is present in the setting of lower back pain (especially in cases of nerve-root compression), it must be considered a likely cause of the symptoms.

Compression of a nerve root may cause loss of strength in the muscles, or loss of sensation in the skin. With long-lasting nerve-root compression, wasting of muscles may also occur. The special X-ray studies described above will usually confirm the clinical suspicion of disk disease.

Even for disk herniation without severe or rapidly progressing symptoms, conservative treatment (bed rest, medication, and special exercises) should be the initial approach. On the other hand, rapid progression of any symptom of paralysis, especially with loss of bowel or bladder control, constitutes an emergency.

In such cases, immediate surgery will likely be recommended.

In the absence of such indications, conservative treatment for at least four to six weeks is the usual procedure. It may be extended for as long as three months, although there is some risk that delaying surgery this long could result in some irreversible damage. Surgery is not routinely recommended in disk disease for two reasons: Conservative therapy often is effective, and the success rate for this kind of surgery is generally unsatisfactory compared to other conditions for which surgery is routinely performed.

The major benefit of surgery is relief of sciatica—virtually complete in about 75 percent of patients, with a diminution of pain in about 90 percent. Relief of lower back pain is less predictable, with complete, long-lasting relief of symptoms expected in only about half the patients who undergo surgery, so this surgery remains controversial.

In view of this, some other procedures have been tried. One of these, **chemonucleolysis**, involves the injection of **chymopapain** (a derivative of the papaya tree) to dissolve sufficient amounts of disk to relieve pressure on the adjacent nerve root. Introduced in 1983, this treatment has gradually fallen out of favor: Long-term results are no better than with conventional surgery, and the procedure has produced some allergic and neurological complications.

If, for whatever reason, surgery does not seem to offer hope of relief or is considered too risky, the road to complete recovery for the patient may be long and difficult. Along with conservative medical therapy, he will need ample amounts of patience and determination. In the absence of dramatic improvement, some patients may turn to alternative, unconventional types of therapy. These may help relieve pain, but, unlike the situation in which no structural disease of the spine is present (chronic nonspecific lower back pain), more harm than good may be accomplished. For example, spinal manipulation as performed by chiropractors is ill-advised and may, on occasion, result in disaster.

How to Prevent Lower Back Pain

Whether or not you have ever suffered from pain in the lower back, you can avoid its occurrence by taking certain preventive measures. For instance, learn the proper way to lift things, especially heavy objects. Don't bend over from the waist when picking up objects on the floor. Instead, squat down by the object, keeping the back straight and the knees bent. Slowly rise with the object. This allows you to use your strong thigh muscles and avoid using your spine as a lever. People who have suffered previous attacks of lower back pain should avoid particular twisting movements or awkward body positions that throw the spine out of alignment.

You can perform a number of safe exercises on a regular basis that will strengthen your back and your abdominal muscles. A good exercise manual or, if you want personal guidance, a sports therapist, can give you advice and suggestions for a daily regimen of such exercises.

Sports Injuries

Participation in sports that involve sudden movements, especially twisting, with or without body contact, is the most frequent cause of muscle and bone injuries. These sports include football, soccer, tennis, baseball, and basketball. Swimming is always recommended as an excellent sport because it is free of such potentially hazardous movements. Recreational running or jogging, although free from the risks of body contact sports, can result in a number of musculoskeletal problems over time. Obviously the likelihood of such injuries is proportional to the number of miles run weekly.

Most of the damage from sports involves the soft tissues, such as muscles and ligaments. Overstretching and/or tearing of these structures is the most common injury. Rest, hot or cold packs, and the use of over-the-counter analgesics usually can manage these minor injuries quite well.

The following are some of the more common sports injuries:

Shin splints. This condition involves the main bone of the lower leg, the tibia. The covering or periosteum becomes inflamed, causing pain and swelling along the inner part of the bone. Runners seem more prone to this than do other types of athletes. Proper warm-up, a gradual increase in the level of exercise, and avoiding hard-surface contact are the best means of prevention.

Tendinitis. This involves inflammation, probably due to sprains or minute calcifications of tendons in various parts of the body. Achilles tendinitis, for example, involves the tendon that inserts into the heel at the back of the foot. Rest and anti-inflammatory medications are recommended. Torn Achilles tendons may require surgery.

Pulled hamstrings. This is a common term referring to over-stretching (strain) of the muscles over the buttocks and back of the thighs.

Tennis elbow. Common in the sport from which it takes its name, tennis elbow is related to repeated stresses on the forearm caused by the rotary motion required for a good tennis topspin. Rest and moist heat can provide relief.

Knee problems. These can occur in a variety of sports in which sudden abnormal or twisting stresses are placed on this joint. Frequently the ligaments supporting and connecting the joint are torn. Blood vessels may be ruptured and bleed into the knee. Cartilaginous structures within the knee, which ordinarily provide additional support and stability, also may become damaged in the course of athletic activity.

In contrast to many other sports injuries, those involving the knee may result in permanent disability unless relieved by surgical intervention. When internal injuries of the knee are severe, X-ray studies, especially arthrograms, can often identify the specific structure involved. Arthroscopy may be required for additional information. As part of the latter procedure, sometimes surgical removal of certain damaged structures is performed to avoid more extensive and complicated surgery of the knee joint.

Dislocations. These are abnormal separations of the bony structures inserting into any of the various joints around the body. They can be relatively minor, involving the fingers, or much more severe, as with dislocations at the shoulder or hip joint. A dislocated joint causes pain, swelling, discoloration, and an inability to move the area. See a doctor as soon as possible.

Charley horse. This refers to a spasm of the muscles, usually in the lower extremities, that may follow excessive stretching of the ligaments involved. Resting the area involved usually helps relieve the pain.

Bursitis. Inflammation of one or more bursae may occur as a result of trauma and excessive activity involving these lubricating sacs. In addition to the usual conservative measures employed for soft-tissue injuries, the injection of cortisone into bursae may provide more rapid and complete relief.

Muscle cramps. These painful, involuntary muscle contractions may be related to sports activity, but also do occur in totally different settings. The ordinary cramp usually begins when a muscle is already in its most shortened position. This may be why swimmers are particularly susceptible to calf cramps: With proper kicking technique in the crawl, the toes are pointed rearward, shortening the calf muscles to the maximum.

A common type is the nocturnal cramp, when the calf muscles may be in a shortened condition as the individual lies in bed, making these muscles more susceptible to spasm. Quinine has been used with questionable benefit to reduce the severity and frequency of these attacks, which are almost always easily terminated by getting out of bed and assuming a standing position to walk and stretch out the muscle.

Stress fractures. In contrast to bone fractures, which result from external trauma, stress fractures are related to repeated muscular action that eventually exceeds the normal bone's ability to maintain its structural integrity. The location of the stress fracture will vary in accordance with the types of activity—stress fractures of the ribs may occur in backpacking, golf, or tennis; the vertebral column may be affected by heavy weightlifting, ballet dancing, or gymnastics; long-distance running can induce such fractures in the long bones of the legs, or in the bones of the feet.

One indication that you might be suffering from a stress fracture is persistent pain in a particular bone when you are performing a specific activity. Often a lump can also be felt over the painful area. Early X rays may miss a stress fracture, although after several weeks of symptoms, a characteristic appearance will become evident. Rest will enable a stress fracture to heal, but recurrences may result from too-early and too-vigorous resumption of the activity that caused them in the first place.

Neurological Conditions Affecting Muscle Function

Nerve activity stimulates muscles to contract. Any disease involving the nerves supplying a particular group of muscles will impair the ability of those muscles to function normally. The nerve structures involved may be located in the central nervous system (brain and spinal cord) or may be more directly aligned with particular muscles; the peripheral nerves in the arms and legs fall into the latter category.

Amyotrophic lateral sclerosis. Also known as Lou Gehrig's disease (from the famous Yankee first baseman who died from it), this is a disease of the motor cells of the spinal cord, those nerve cells that supply the fibers responsible for motion and other muscle activities. A relatively rare neurological disease, it usually appears in midlife or later years. The cause is unknown, the treatment merely supportive, and the outcome always fatal some years after the diagnosis has been made.

Multiple sclerosis. This is a disease of young adults and much more common than amyotrophic lateral sclerosis. In the northern part of the United States, between 30 and 80 individuals for every 100,000 are affected. It is much less common in southern climes and virtually nonexistent in the tropics. The cause is unknown. A virus has been suspected but never proven responsible. It is called a **demyelinating disease** because it involves the destruction of the myelin sheaths that enclose the nerve fibers in the brain and spinal cord.

People who develop multiple sclerosis characteristically experience certain symptoms that eventually resolve to some degree spontaneously only to recur at a later time—the pattern of "exacerbation and remission" referred to by neurologists. Symptoms may involve sudden weakness of a set of muscles, blurriness or loss of vision, unsteadiness of gait, or loss of urinary or bowel control.

There is no clear-cut laboratory test for multiple sclerosis, and the initial symptoms may be slight. Physicians do not make the diagnosis of multiple sclerosis lightly because of its ultimately poor prognosis. While there is no cure, physical therapy can help to control symptoms.

Guillain-Barré syndrome. After certain viral infections, such as a bout of influenza, some individuals develop a fatigue or general body weakness beginning in the limbs and progressing upward throughout the body. This weakness eventually may result in complete paralysis requiring mechanical ventilators to support breathing, and tube-feeding for nutrition. This disorder, called Guillain-Barré syndrome, may involve the myelin sheaths of peripheral nerves or the central nervous system.

Despite its occasionally life-threatening nature, the disease is usually self-limiting. With adequate supportive treatment, complete recovery occurs over time in the majority of those affected.

Carpal tunnel syndrome. Carpal tunnel syndrome results from nerve compression at the wrist, where the nerve supplying the muscles of the thumb and adjacent two or three fingers passes through a tunnel formed by fibrous tissue. Any tissue or fluid accumulation in this narrow tunnel can put pressure on this nerve, causing symptoms of numbness and tingling. These sensations often occur at night, with accompanying pain. Gradually the muscles of the thumb and palm may atrophy or waste away.

The causes of this syndrome are many, and include rheumatoid arthritis, thyroid disease, and diabetes. Each cause requires specific treatment. Immediate therapy involves relief of the pressure by local injection of steroids or, in severe cases, surgical relief of the obstruction.

Peripheral neuropathy. Any disease involving the peripheral nerves can affect associated muscle functions. Peripheral neuropathy, which may be irreversible, can occur in a variety of settings and for a variety of reasons, including chemical poisoning (arsenic, mercury, lead), alcoholism, and diabetes.

2

The Healthy Heart

Heart disease, primarily coronary heart disease, remains the major cause of death among American men, despite a gratifying decrease in its incidence over the past few years. Each year nearly five and half million Americans are diagnosed as having coronary heart disease and it causes over a half-million deaths in this country. Although following menopause women begin to catch up with men, the much higher incidence of coronary disease in men during the middle and later decades of their lives—their prime years in terms of family, business, and society—makes heart disease a particularly male malady.

One exception to this is valvular heart disease, which affects both men and women equally. Fortunately, valvular heart disease resulting from rheumatic fever has decreased considerably in the United States over the past two decades. Rheumatic fever comes about as a reaction of the body's immune system to an earlier streptococcal infection; thus many specialists believe that aggressive treatment with antibiotics of all suspected "strep throats" has led to this decline. There are other categories of valve disease, congenital and acquired, but these make up a small percentage of the cardiac problems seen in this country.

The heart is a muscle, and it stands to reason that most heart disease involves this muscle. But for a long time we have known that diseases of the blood vessels, particularly of the arteries supplying the heart with blood, can be found as either underlying or contributing causes of most heart disease, so much so that this general category of pathology is referred to as **coronary artery disease** (CAD). Now there is an increasing awareness that cardiomyopathies, diseases directly affecting the heart muscle itself, can play a role in many of the problems we had previously thought of as cardiovascular.

THE HEART AT WORK

The human heart is essentially a four-chambered pump (see Figure 2.1). The two chambers on the right, called the **right atrium** and **right ventricle**, receive dark red blood returning through the veins from various parts of the body where our muscles and organs have extracted oxygen to do their normal work. From the right side of the heart, blood is pumped via the **pulmonary artery** to the lungs for oxygenation and then through the **pulmonary veins** to the other two chambers, first the **left atrium** and then the **left ventricle**. This bright red blood, now carrying its full complement of oxygen, is ejected by the left ventricle through the vessel arising from it, the **aorta**, to the various tissues of the body.

Valves located strategically within this four-chambered system prevent the blood from flowing backward when the ventricles contract. Between the right atrium and right ventricle the **tricuspid valve**, so called because of its three-cusp structure, performs that function. The two-cusped **mitral valve**, named for its resemblance to a bishop's miter, does identical duty between the left atrium and left ventricle. Jointly, the mitral and tricuspid valves are referred to as the **atrioventricular** (or AV) valves.

With each contraction of the ventricles, the blood passes into a major vessel: the pulmonary artery arising from the right ventricle, the aorta arising from the left ventricle. As the ventricles relax after each contraction, a set of symmetrical three-cusped

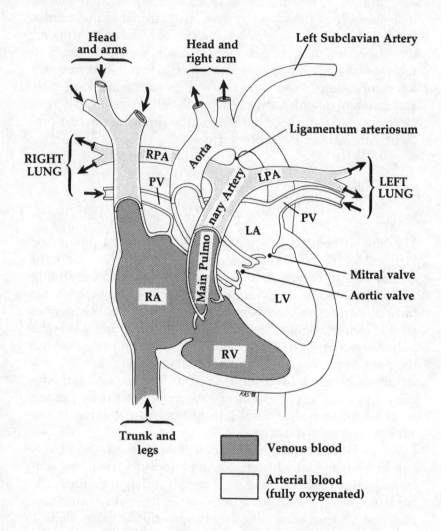

Figure 2.1   The heart and its major vessels

(or semilunar) valves prevent blood from flowing backward into the ventricles. These are the **pulmonic** and **aortic** valves.

The **pericardium** (not shown in Figure 2.1) is a thin-walled but sturdy sac in which the heart is enclosed within the chest. The sac contains a small amount of fluid that probably provides lubrication between the surfaces of the heart and the pericardium.

Like the rest of the body, the heart depends upon an oxygen supply to meet its great needs for continuous functioning. While the body as a whole may extract only 25 to 35 percent of the oxygen contained in the arterial blood delivered to it, the heart ordinarily extracts close to 65 percent. To satisfy the needs of this constantly working pump, two major vessels branch out of the aorta as it emerges from the left ventricle (see Figure 2.2). They "sit" above the heart, giving rise to various branches that cover the heart's suface before plunging through the walls to the deeper layers of heart muscle. Hence the term *coronary*, from the Latin word for "crown" or "garland," to describe the right and left coronary arteries.

Cardiac output is a common measure of heart performance. Usually expressed on a per-minute basis, the cardiac output can be calculated from the heart rate and volume of blood ejected with each heartbeat. The normal heart rate at rest varies between 60 and 100 beats per minute, the volume of blood pumped by the ventricles varying accordingly to give a normal cardiac output of about five liters (1.3 gallons) per minute in a normal-sized man. With exercise or other stress, this rate can double or, in some people, even triple.

Making the Diagnosis

To a remarkable degree, evaluation of the health of the heart can be gauged quite accurately by a physician in his or her office. With no more information than that provided by age and sex, symptoms, a physical examination, and, usually, a resting electrocardiogram or ECG (see below), an astute physician can make an accurate estimation of whether or not the problem is cardiac in nature and, if so, what might be the type and extent of the disorder.

When this initial evaluation does not suffice, a number of

External view showing the right and left coronary arteries
arising from the aorta to distribute blood to the heart muscle.

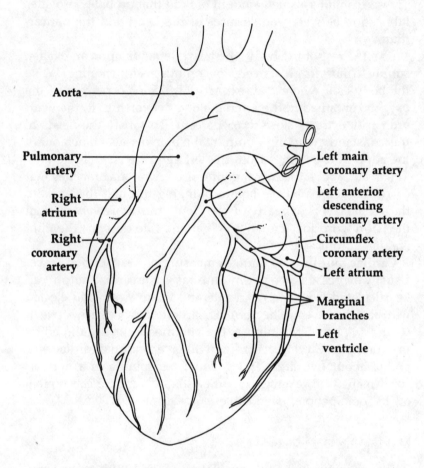

Figure 2.2   External view of the heart

other diagnostic methods can be used. Most of these tests are painless, without significant risk, and easily performed on an outpatient basis. With them, a physician can almost invariably uncover the problem.

Electrocardiography (ECG). The resting ECG (also known as an EKG) remains the standard test for diagnosing many of the potential abnormalities that may affect the heart. An ECG is a tracing of the minute waves of electrical activity that spread from the atria to the ventricles to stimulate muscular contractions. It is used to determine heart rate and to detect extra heartbeats arising in various parts of the heart, excessive slowing or racing of the heart, and abnormal or disturbed conduction of activating impulses within the heart. The ECG can also suggest the enlargement or thickening of a heart chamber. It can detect damage to the heart muscle that may occur when a coronary artery is blocked, or even a transient lack of blood flow that has not progressed to destruction of heart muscle. An ECG may also indicate inflammation of the pericardium.

Treadmill testing. Several variations on the standard ECG have become incorporated into modern diagnosis. Although a person with coronary artery disease may have a normal ECG while at rest, evidence of inadequate blood supply to the heart muscle, called **ischemia**, may become apparent on an ECG taken during exercise. For this purpose, treadmill testing with electrocardiographic monitoring can prove useful in evaluating chest pain to determine whether it is caused by insufficiency of coronary flow.

The test is simple. You walk on a treadmill and, by increasing its slope and speed, the physician attempts to make you gradually increase your exercise to a "target" heart rate. In other words, the heart is placed at a stress level that is adequate to uncover evidence on the ECG of inadequate coronary blood flow.

There are two major concerns about such testing: safety and accuracy. When performed with the proper indications (for example, the evaluation of chest pain) and under the guidance of an experienced physician, studies of treadmill testing performed among hundreds of thousands of patients have found that death has resulted in only three to ten patients per hundred thousand. In view of the fact that such patients are selected because the presence of coronary heart disease is suspected, in the main this slight risk should be considered acceptable. Any person about to undergo such testing may confidently approach it without fear of dire results.

In terms of reliability or dependability of the test, two types of errors may occur: false positives and false negatives—respectively, the appearance of ECG abnormalities in normal patients and the failure of ECG changes to appear in patients with coronary heart disease. The reliability of the test varies with the type of patient or population studied. For example, it predicts quite well the presence or absence of coronary disease in middle-aged men, a group with a relatively high prevalence of coronary disease. Among other groups—such as women, younger men, and those with resting ECG abnormalities—the test is less reliable.

Radioactive tracers. When results of regular stress testing are inconclusive, or if the doctor anticipates problems of interpretation, treadmill testing can be combined with the intravenous injection into the bloodstream of a small amount of the radioactive tracer **thallium**. The image of the tracer in the blood is revealed by a special scanner that follows the course of blood flow to the heart muscle. In this way, treadmill testing is made more sensitive to certain abnormalities, and avoids false positive ECG results in some patients.

Holter monitoring. This is an application of the ECG named after the physician who pioneered the technique. Electrodes are applied to the skin with adhesive. These lead to a device similar to a tape recorder that records the heart rate and rhythm over a preselected period, usually 24 hours, to detect variations in heart rate and any unusual beats that may occur during this time. More recently, improved types of Holter monitoring have been able to record other findings in the ECG indicative of inadequate blood supply to the heart. The patient can also keep a simple diary in which he notes any symptoms during this time. When the tape is returned to the physician or monitoring station, the 24-hour record can be quickly scanned for abnormalities, some of which the patient may be unaware of as well as any that coincide with his symptoms.

Other devices. If symptoms occur less frequently, there are electronic devices that can be placed against a telephone as the patient holds the wire leads in his armpits. The ECG record can be made from information telephonically transmitted to a receiving station. In this way, rarely occurring symptoms and irregularities of the heart may be documented.

X-ray studies. In the past, aside from physical examination, which often missed early changes, the chest X ray was the only means of detecting enlargement of the heart. Although it is still somewhat useful for this purpose, it has been largely supplanted by cardiac ultrasound (see below). Today the main value of the chest X ray in cardiac patients is its display of lungs that may have become congested. An X ray can also detect fluid in the space between the lungs and chest wall, known as **pleural effusion**, which can occur in heart failure. Of course, cardiac patients are as susceptible to pneumonias, lung tumors, and other lung problems as the rest of us, and for these purposes the chest X ray remains valuable.

MUGA scan. Other radiological studies have assumed major importance in the evaluation of heart patients. These techniques involve injecting radioactive substances into an arm vein and, shortly afterwards, using a scanner or scope to visualize the heart, either at rest or during exercise. The common term for studies outlining the heart chambers and showing the motion of its walls is MUGA, for multigated scan. Thallium is the agent used for "myocardial perfusion" studies, which show the distribution of blood flow within the heart muscle walls themselves. For examination of the heart chambers, technetium is the agent ordinarily used. Both types of study can be performed in association with exercise. Since these tests involve only injection of material into an arm vein, they are still classified as noninvasive, in contrast to cardiac catheterization (see below).

CT scans and MR imaging. The relatively new X-ray technique of computed tomography, or CT scanning, has some applications in diagnosing heart disease. The images produced actually appear as anatomical sections through the chest. The even newer technique of magnetic resonance imaging, or MRI, has greater potential for cardiac diagnosis. The images are similar to those produced by CT scanning, but are often of higher quality and are better suited for evaluation of the heart structure.

In MRI, magnetic fields rather than X rays are used to produce an image. Using "gating" techniques—photographically stopping the heart motion at any point in its cycle—some remarkable images have been obtained.

Cardiac ultrasound (echocardiography). At this time, neither CT scanning nor MRI offers the ease, economy, and variety of information obtained by cardiac ultrasound. The use of sound waves to explore the structure of the heart has become the laboratory mainstay in the noninvasive approach to cardiac diagnosis. Painlessly, and without any side effects, sound waves pass through the heart when a transducer is applied to the chest wall in a space between two ribs. The echoes reflected from the surfaces of the heart can be recorded in a number of ways. Originally, in **moving-mode** (or M-mode) **echocardiography**, only an "icepick" of sound could be employed, producing a number of wavy lines on the recording paper decipherable only by a trained echocardiographer. Later, **two-dimensional** (or 2-D) **echocardiography** was able to produce on a monitor anatomically correct images showing the heart beating. With these two techniques combined, physicians can obtain accurate dimensions of the heart, detect valvular abnormalities and abnormalities of wall motion, and spot tumors, clots, and fluid around the heart within the pericardial space. The heart's functional status can also be ascertained easily.

M-mode and 2-D echocardiography are ultrasonic techniques, which means the sound employed is beyond the range of human hearing. These have now been supplemented by **Doppler echocardiography**, in which audible sound reflected from blood coursing through the heart can be used to detect normal and abnormal flow patterns. In some cases the velocities of these flow patterns can actually be used to predict pressures within the heart. Color-coded Doppler produces images that reflect in vivid hues the flow of blood within the cardiac chambers.

The latest innovation in cardiac ultrasound is **transesophageal echocardiography**. In some patients the images obtained from placing the pickup device on the chest wall are of such poor quality as to be useless. In others, certain important structures of the heart cannot be visualized by the conventional approach. Since the esophagus runs directly behind the heart, excellent images of the heart can be obtained from a transducer mounted on an endoscope that you are able to swallow. First a local anesthetic is sprayed on the back of your throat and you are usually sedated intravenously. Although this procedure can hardly be considered noninvasive and you may experience some discomfort, it can be performed quickly (in 10 to 20 minutes), is safe, and can provide invaluable information to your physician.

Cardiac catheterization. The invasive procedure of cardiac catheterization involves the introduction of long, flexible tubes into an arm or leg vein or artery (or both) and snaking these catheters into the right and left sides of the heart respectively. Cardiologists are then able to measure directly the pressures in the heart and blood vessels, take blood samples to determine oxygen content, and measure cardiac output. They also inject radiopaque dye into the heart chambers and coronary arteries, and take motion pictures of the radiographic images to reveal abnormalities of heart structure and function. This discipline is called **cineangiography**.

In the 1940s and 1950s, as surgical techniques became available to correct many congenital and acquired heart diseases (the latter mainly valvular in nature), cardiac catheterization became essential so that the surgeon would know precisely his or her task before the operation. Today most of this information can be obtained noninvasively, primarily by echocardiography.

The one part of heart structure currently beyond the reach of echocardiography and other noninvasive techniques is delineation of the coronary arteries. As coronary artery disease gained recognition as a major problem among American men, and coronary bypass surgery (see page 59) was shown to be a generally effective treatment, this type of cardiac catheterization became the primary indicator of coronary artery disease in adult men.

HYPERTENSION

In its several degrees of severity, high blood pressure (or hypertension) affects approximately 60 million Americans.

High blood pressure is a major cause of concern because it can result directly in heart disease, called **hypertensive cardiovascular disease**, or promote the development of coronary heart disease. It may also damage other organs within the body, primarily the brain and kidneys. Fortunately, despite its high prevalence in our country and its serious consequences for health and even survival, it can usually be controlled by currently available methods.

Each time the left ventricle pumps part of its contents into the arterial system, the introduction of new blood in this series of tubes causes the pressure to rise. The peak pressure achieved is called **systolic**. As the left ventricle relaxes, the aortic valve closes to prevent any backflow of blood into the ventricle. As the blood that has been ejected into the arterial system finds its way into the capillaries and veins, the pressure within the arteries falls. The lowest pressure reached before the next contraction is called **diastolic**. The levels of both systolic and diastolic blood pressure are what the physician or nurse measures in the office. They are expressed in millimeters of mercury to correspond to the height of the mercury column in the blood-pressure measuring apparatus, which is called a **sphygmomanometer**.

Besides the volume of blood ejected with each beat, the pressure developed in the arteries depends on other factors: the thickness of the blood, lesser in anemia, greater in polycythemia; the composition of the arterial walls, more elastic in children, stiffer in adults; and the total blood volume in the body. Alcohol, nicotine, caffeine, and undue excitement and stress can also raise blood pressure, the system being very sensitive to all types of nervous and hormonal stimulation.

Among normal adults, the general upper limits listed for normal blood pressure are 140 millimeters of mercury for systolic pressure and 90 for diastolic pressure; this is generally written as 140/90. *Mild* hypertension is defined by a diastolic pressure ranging between 90 and 104. *Moderate* hypertension is defined by diastolic pressures between 105 and 114. Diastolic readings of 115 and above fall into the category of *severe* hypertension. **Isolated systolic hypertension** exists when the systolic pressure is over 160 millimeters of mercury while the diastolic pressure is within the normal range.

Low Blood Pressure

With most human disorders, every extreme at one end of the scale has a corresponding illness at the other—hyperthyroidism and hypothyroidism, anemia and polycythemia, and so forth. In practical terms, however, this does not hold for blood pressure. Of course, people bleeding to death, or those with severe injuries or bloodstream infections, and victims of massive heart attacks may have precipitous drops in blood pressure resulting in shock. But, in general, there is no chronic illness involving abnormally low blood pressure.

Despite this, many people are concerned about having chronically low blood pressure. If you are among them, keep in mind that there is no sharp dividing line between low, normal, and high blood pressure. The defined limits, even for high blood pressure, are somewhat arbitrary, and your "low" pressure simply signifies that you are fortunate in having arteries much younger than your chronological age. The lower your blood pressure, the better off you are. Those people at 100/70 are most likely at less risk for coronary problems than are those at 120/80, who are better off than those at 135/88—yet all of these readings fall within the defined "normal" range.

Causes of Hypertension

Hypertension may be defined as "secondary" or "curable" in cases where some specific abnormality that is usually correctable by surgery can be identified. Certain tumors can cause hypertension. Narrowing of an artery supplying a kidney, called **renal artery stenosis**, is another form of hypertensive disease that can be surgically corrected. Some people are born with a severe narrowing of the aorta just beyond the branch that supplies blood to the head and arms. As a result, these people have high pressure when measured in the arms, with lower readings when measured in the legs. This type of narrowing can be corrected by surgery as well.

If the patient is young and has high blood pressure, or if he has very severe hypertension that does not seem to respond well to therapy, these disorders must be considered among its potential causes, and the necessary diagnostic investigations should be undertaken. But in the vast majority of people with high blood pressure—about 95 percent—no identifiable, specific cause is likely to be found, and extensive diagnostic work-ups are unnecessary. Hypertension with no known cause is termed "essential hypertension."

Symptoms of Hypertension

Essential hypertension usually appears after the age of thirty. Although in the past certain symptoms were believed to be associated with high blood pressure—nosebleeds, headaches, dizziness—recent studies of people with hypertension, compared against controls with normal blood pressure, have revealed no significant differences in the incidence of these problems between the two groups. On the contrary, most people with high blood pressure feel perfectly well until one of the complications of their disease results in a possibly serious illness. For this reason, periodic physical examinations with blood pressure measurements are important, especially among those who come from families with a history of hypertension.

Diagnosis of Hypertension

The diagnosis of moderate or severe hypertension can usually be made accurately in the doctor's office. A therapeutic program can then be undertaken. When a doctor detects only mild hypertension on a single measurement, it is important to ascertain that this is a consistent finding and not related only to the excitement of the moment as the doctor applies the blood pressure cuff. To obtain a proper baseline, the physician should allow at least five to 10 minutes of relaxation before measuring blood pressure. The patient should avoid caffeine and smoking for at least an hour or two before the examination.

No diagnosis of mild hypertension should be made unless it is confirmed on two or more visits to the doctor's office. At times, even this will not suffice. "White coat hypertension," the elevation of blood pressure only when the doctor measures it, has been documented in cases when the nurses or office assistants consistently get normal pressures while on the same visits the doctor is recording higher ones.

The physical examination of hypertensives, other than that involved in taking the blood pressure, is often unrevealing. With the ophthalmoscope the physician may occasionally detect changes at the back of the eye due to hypertension, but even when the heart has been moderately enlarged by long-standing hypertension, the doctor may be unable to detect enlargement without resorting to X-ray or ultrasonic examination.

Effects of Hypertension

Chronic elevations of blood pressure can result in damage to several organ systems. The wall of the left ventricle of the heart may thicken first. Later this chamber may dilate as the heart fails in its attempts to maintain its output against such high pressure. Congestive heart failure (see page 57) may ultimately ensue if no antihypertensive treatment is given.

The presence of hypertension also promotes the development of coronary artery disease. The complications of coronary disease may actually result in the first symptoms that the patient experiences.

Severe elevation of blood pressure may result in strokes, either from bleeding or from clots forming in the vessels of the brain. The strokes destroy vital nerve cells in the affected areas. The main vessel leading from the left heart, the aorta, may develop weakness and tears with catastrophic consequences. Chronic hypertension can also damage the kidney tissues; some people with kidneys damaged in this way go on to complete kidney failure and require regular hemodialysis sessions to maintain their life thereafter.

Treatment of Hypertension

There is no question about the need to treat moderate and severe hypertension. In certain cases deemed **hypertensive emergencies**, when abrupt, severe elevations of blood pressure may be life-threatening, hospitalization may even be necessary to bring the patient's blood pressure under control. Some controversy exists about the need to treat people with mild hypertension. The benefits of therapy in these cases have been less demonstrable than in the more severe forms. The current trend, however, has been strongly in favor of treatment. Recently, isolated systolic hypertension, which is more common among older people and has often been neglected in the past, has received increased attention, with a similar shift in attitudes toward favoring therapy to prevent complications.

Non-drug methods. In the presence of hypertension, especially when mild, certain alterations in life-style and habits may prove effective in lowering blood pressure. Avoiding alcohol and stopping smoking may bring pressures down to within the normal range. Among the overweight, slimming down can have a significant effect upon blood pressure. Regular exercise may not only help reduce weight but lower blood pressure as well.

The majority of the public, and even some health professionals, generally believe that excessive salt intake plays a major role in hypertension. Actually, the connection between salt and high blood pressure tends to be exaggerated. Although most Americans ingest much more sodium in the form of salt than their bodies need, in only about 30 percent of white hypertensives does salt intake seem to affect blood pressure. The figure for African Americans is slightly higher, at 45 percent. Since there is no easy way of readily determining who among hypertensive patients is sensitive, the general approach is to restrict salt and see what effect this has on blood pressure.

Behavior modification involving biofeedback and relaxation exercises can be effective in lowering blood pressure, but these techniques have not achieved wide usage, probably because of the greater convenience in prescribing one of the many effective drugs currently available for treatment of hypertension. For the motivated person, however, such techniques, along with smoking cessation, severely restricting alcohol, weight loss, and exercise, may eliminate the need for medications and their possible side effects.

Drug therapy. When non-drug methods fail to control blood pressure, a variety of medications at the disposal of the physician almost always will do the job. Most experience has been accumulated with diuretics, sometimes known as "water pills," which, when taken as the sole agent, control blood pressure in as many as 85 percent of patients by decreasing the volume of blood in the arteries and veins. A "stepped-care" approach has been advocated for people more resistant to treatment. Another type of drug and, less often, a third can be added to bring blood pressure under control. It is a rare patient who will not respond to such a regimen.

Medications other than diuretics include **beta blockers, vasodilators, calcium channel blockers**, and the recently introduced **angiotensin converting enzyme (ACE) inhibitors.**

Currently, selection of the best first drug is undergoing reexamination. Diuretics, for example, do not reverse thickening of the heart's walls even when blood pressure is controlled. And they may adversely affect blood lipid levels. For these reasons, and because long-term studies have failed to show dramatic improvement in the coronary complications of people treated with diuretics, other medications are undergoing scrutiny as more appropriate to begin therapy. Every drug has the potential to cause side effects. Aside from occasional rashes and other allergic reactions, patients using one or more of these drugs may experience drowsiness, lethargy, fatigue, breathing difficulties, dizziness, fainting, and, of special importance to men, impotence.

Because so many people with high blood pressure feel so much better when off their medication, even with uncontrolled, elevated blood-pressure levels, there is a tendency for some men to discontinue medication or reduce doses on their own whenever troubling side effects appear. If you are undergoing treatment for hypertension, it is much wiser to discuss any suspected unpleasant drug effects with your doctor and to participate with the doctor in the selection of the best drug for you. *Do not change your medical regimen without medical consultation and guidance.* This is one of the medical situations in which how you feel is *not* your best guide.

Fortunately, drug treatment for hypertension need not be a lifelong sentence. In multiple studies of hypertensive patients whose blood pressure was kept within the normal range for a year or more, withdrawal of medication did not always result in subsequent pressure elevations. From 15 to as high as 75 percent of the patients continued to show normal readings after medication was discontinued. In such people, it seems that drug therapy reset the body's blood-pressure-control mechanisms to lower levels. People exhibiting this effect should, however, continue to have their blood pressure monitored regularly for evidence of recurring hypertension.

CORONARY ARTERY DISEASE

Coronary artery disease (CAD) is the result of a progressive change, called **atherosclerosis**, within the walls of the coronary arteries. In this disease the cells of the inner lining of the arteries proliferate, and as this occurs, fat is deposited in the walls as well. As the mixture of the cells and fat accumulates along the walls, the mass or **plaque** protrudes into the passageway (or lumen) of the artery, interfering with the free flow of blood supplying the heart muscle. At some point, atherosclerotic plaque may gradually close off the vessel. More often there is a sudden blockage (or occlusion) caused by a rupture of the plaque followed by a blood clot forming on the surface of the plaque. This is the scenario in what is commonly termed a heart attack or, more precisely, an **acute coronary occlusion with myocardial infarction**.

The medical consequence is that the heart muscle is damaged by the loss of its blood supply. Although people frequently speak of "heart attack," the term is not specific enough to be useful for interpretation by doctors trying to treat the problem. What a patient describes as a heart attack may truly be a myocardial infarction. But at other times the patient may be describing any of the many symptoms—shortness of breath, palpitations, chest pain—that do sometimes, but not always, indicate that there has been a sufficient deprivation of blood to the heart to cause heart-muscle damage.

Angina

Angina, or angina pectoris, is a particular, intermittent pain or pressure felt in the chest by patients with coronary heart problems when increased needs of the heart for oxygen cannot be met. At rest, the patient may be able to maintain an adequate blood supply to the heart muscle. But under conditions of physical stress, such as exercise, an increase in flow adequate to meet the demands of the heart muscle may be unattainable. This lack of oxygen-containing blood flow to the heart, called **ischemia**, results in chest pain that may also travel to the arms (particularly the left arm) or the jaw.

Angina can occur in other situations that ordinarily give rise to increased demands for blood flow and oxygen supply such as excitement, anxiety, and aggravation. Transient increases in blood pressure may tip the balance of a limited coronary reserve toward angina, since the heart has to work harder to pump against increased pressures and resistance in the arteries. Rapid heart rates may induce angina because the oxygen requirement over each minute of time is proportional to the number of beats occurring within that period. (Walking against a cold wind, for example, frequently provokes angina.) Finally, anemia may cause angina in coronary artery disease because of the decreased oxygen content in each drop of blood owing to the scarcity of red cells.

The pain of angina caused by artery disease usually lasts no more than 15 to 20 minutes, and is relieved by rest or antianginal drugs such as nitroglycerine (see below).

Angina does not always signify coronary artery obstruction. Severe hypertension alone may result in a thickened muscle wall that the coronary arteries cannot supply with an adequate amount of blood. A similar imbalance may occur when the opening of the aortic valve narrows, which leads to increased thickness, or **hypertrophy**, of the left ventricle. Occasionally, with or without underlying atherosclerosis, the coronary artery may go into spasm, causing angina or even myocardial infarction. This may be the mechanism that causes ischemia in cocaine users and others with no apparent cause for chest pain. Finally, the blood platelets, whose function is to initiate clotting, may promote the formation of small aggregates of blood cells that form and disperse periodically, resulting in anginal symptoms due to intermittent obstruction of blood flow.

Recently, **silent angina** has received increased attention. In the evaluation of coronary patients, prolonged ECG monitoring has revealed marked, fluctuating ischemia of which the patient is completely unaware. The persistence of these episodes during a 24-hour period of monitoring has been shown to be related to an increased incidence of myocardial infarction later on.

Treatment. Patients with angina of mild or moderate severity that has not changed its pattern over many months (**chronic stable angina**) benefit the most from drug therapy. This approach aims at reducing those factors that lead to greater demands of the heart muscle for oxygen.

Antianginal drug medication includes, as its cornerstone, nitrates such as **nitroglycerine** preparations or nitroglycerine-containing patches that are worn on the skin, or the longer-acting **isosorbide dinitrate** (Isordil or Sorbitrate). Beta blockers such as **metoprolol** (Lopressor) or **atenolol** (Tenormin) may be added to the drug regimen for additional control, although calcium-channel blockers such as **nifedipine** (Procardia), **diltiazem** (Cardizem), and **verapamil** (Calan) may prove at least as useful as the beta blockers in this regard and perhaps with fewer side effects.

Unstable angina is indicated when the symptoms have suddenly become more prolonged and severe, often when the patient is at rest. Patients are admitted to the hospital for the administration of drugs, as well as for anticoagulation therapy with **heparin** or aspirin. As soon as such attacks are under control, physicians often perform coronary arteriography to determine whether surgery or angioplasty (see page 62) is needed to relieve the condition.

Myocardial Infarction

This is a more severe stage of the disease, in which prolonged lack of blood supply to the heart muscle results in the destruction of the tissue (infarction). Although the episode may be painless or produce only minor discomfort in about 20 percent of such cases—these are known as "silent" infarctions—most victims experience severe, prolonged chest pain.

Unlike angina, the pain of an acute myocardial infarction usually lasts for several hours and is unrelieved by either rest or the usual doses of antianginal medication. As noted above, in almost all cases of acute myocardial infarction, the underlying process involves the sudden formation of a **thrombus**, or blood clot, on atherosclerotic plaque in the arteries.

Treatment. Therapy for an infarction has two goals: to limit the amount of damage to the heart muscle, and to prevent cardiac arrest owing to the lethal arrhythmias that may follow the event.

An electrocardiogram, taken on the patient's admission to the hospital, frequently can diagnose an ongoing episode of myocardial infarction. Blood work can confirm the diagnosis; as the heart muscle is damaged, it releases certain enzymes into the bloodstream. A rise in the levels of these enzymes over the first three days after the event will confirm the ECG findings, or provide evidence of infarction when the ECG is unclear. The degree to which the enzyme levels become elevated can give the examining physician a general idea of the extent of the damage to the patient's heart. Echocardiography and certain nuclear medicine studies may also help to make the diagnosis, especially in confusing or unusual cases.

Ventricular arrhythmias pose a major threat in acute myocardial infarction. These are extra heartbeats arising in the ventricles of the heart, and they may increase in number and intensity to the point where the heart is in **ventricular fibrillation**. In this state the heart is beating so rapidly and in such an uncoordinated manner that it cannot effectively pump blood; if visualized, the heart resembles a bag of squirming worms. This condition or, more rarely, complete cessation of the heartbeat are the two forms of cardiac arrest encountered in infarction patients. The use of antiarrhythmic drugs during the first few days, as the patients are observed in intensive care units, usually prevents the onset of such life-threatening arrhythmias. When they do occur, electrically charged paddles can be placed on the chest; the jolt of current rapidly restores the rhythm to normal. As a result of such measures, the death rate from acute myocardial infarction in hospitals has been halved, from about 30 to less than 15 percent.

If patients are seen early enough, the process of myocardial infarction can be substantially reversed by the intravenous administration of clot-dissolving medication. One of these is the enzyme **streptokinase**; the other is **tissue plasminogen activator** (t-PA). (Newer drugs that are possibly more effective or safer, or both, are currently being evaluated.) This form of therapy is called **thrombolysis**. Its effectiveness in preserving the heart muscle is directly related to the speed with which physicians can initiate treatment to dissolve the clots and restore the flow

Aspirin Therapy

Blood clotting plays a prominent role in the origins and progression of cardiovascular disease. To prevent clotting, various drugs that affect blood coagulation have been tried; surprisingly, the most accessible of all—aspirin—has emerged as one of the most useful in this respect.

Clotting happens when tiny blood platelets within the coronary vessels adhere to each other. Aspirin reduces the stickiness of the platelets, thus preventing clot formation. When tested among those who had already suffered their first myocardial infarction, aspirin was shown to reduce the likelihood of subsequent infarctions. Results of a nationwide study conducted among physicians demonstrated that, among men aged 50 or above who had no previous history of coronary problems, aspirin reduced the incidence of first myocardial infarction by almost one-half.

The decision to take aspirin regularly for the purpose of heart-disease prevention is a personal one. Although aspirin has a long record of safety in general, it does have some side effects in certain people. Some people experience significant gastrointestinal bleeding when they take aspirin; others cannot tolerate it because of increased stomach distress of one sort or another. People with uncontrolled hypertension, among others, may suffer an increased rate of brain hemorrhages after taking aspirin regularly for long periods.

For those who do choose to take aspirin as a preventative, the usual dosage is one standard aspirin tablet every other day.

of blood to the heart. Best results are obtained when thrombolysis is begun within two hours after chest pains start. After four to six hours of symptoms, the usefulness of thrombolysis is markedly diminished, and it is therefore usually not recommended.

After a patient survives an acute myocardial infarction, the uppermost questions in his mind are often, "Am I going to have another attack? If so, when?" Most patients who suffer another attack do so within three to six months following the first. One approach to reducing risk of future attacks would be to perform heart catheterizations on *all* patients soon after their first myocardial infarction, to find those at highest risk. But this is an extremely expensive approach that is also impractical and not without its own risk, given the small but definite complication rate of heart catheterization.

By checking for certain clinical characteristics in patients with myocardial infarction and performing limited specialized testing, such as Holter monitoring and modified treadmill exercise testing, cardiologists can identify those people with the greatest likelihood for future trouble, and proceed to study them further by catheterization. X-ray motion pictures of heart-wall motion can then be performed, and those patients most suitable for bypass surgery or angioplasty can then be selected.

Sudden Death and Congestive Heart Failure

Another manifestation of coronary artery disease is **sudden death**. It may even be the first and last symptom for as many as 30 percent of coronary patients. Some confusion exists as to its definition and various causes. When termed "instantaneous," or occurring within minutes, sudden death is almost always related to coronary heart disease. Death occurring within an hour to two after symptoms start can also be attributed to CAD about 80 to 90 percent of the time. In patients developing sudden chest pains or other symptoms possibly related to the cardiovascular system, and then succumbing within a 24-hour period, autopsy studies have revealed underlying CAD to be the cause in about 60 percent of cases.

Sudden death in CAD may be related to one of two events: a full-blown coronary occlusion with myocardial infarction, or lethal arrhythmias triggered by other reductions in coronary blood flow. Lethal arrhythmias may be related to a spasm narrowing a coronary artery or to incompletely formed blood clots that form and break up, but not before causing temporary obstruction and terminal irregularities of the heartbeat. The ventricles may beat in such a rapid and uncoordinated way as to pump ineffectively, a condition called fibrillation, or simply cease to beat at all, which is called **asystole**. In either event, the patient is unconscious and in **cardiac arrest**.

In those who have complained of chest pain for some hours preceding the cardiac arrest, an underlying myocardial infarction is likely to be found at autopsy. In those in whom the event is even more sudden, one of the other mechanisms usually explains the death.

Congestive heart failure represents a syndrome that may be the end result of a number of types of heart disease. All have in common the inability of the remaining viable heart muscle to perform its functions adequately. In CAD, owing to the loss of significant amounts of functional muscle as a result of previous myocardial infarction—usually more than one—the scar tissue formed as a result has no pumping capacity and the remaining viable heart muscle finds the task beyond its capabilities.

Heart failure can be described as left-sided or right-sided. Failing chambers of the left heart produce primarily symptoms of shortness of breath, inability to lie flat, and congestion of the lungs as revealed by physical examination and chest X ray. When the right side of the heart fails, the symptoms are more often related to accumulation of fluid in the pleural and abdominal cavities, with congestion of the liver and other organs accompanied by edema (swelling) of the lower extremities. Frequently, left- and right-heart failure appear together, and in both cases fatigue may also be a prominent symptom. In CAD, symptoms of left-heart failure usually appear first, but are often followed by right-heart failure as well.

Treatment. The risk of sudden, unexpected death among CAD patients is related to the frequency and severity of ventricular arrhythmias, which can be detected by 24 hours of Holter monitoring after the immediate danger period is over. Treatment to prevent sudden death from ventricular fibrillation has been frustrating, however. Most of the drugs used to suppress these extra beats can potentially incite them as well, even when administered in doses considered within the normal range. Additionally, some of the drugs have severe side effects.

Both of the above considerations have dampened initial enthusiasm for the routine use of such drugs, and the search goes on for a better antiarrhythmic medication. Fortunately, ventricular function is a much stronger predictor of future attacks than is the rhythmic pattern. Except for the most severe arrhythmias, troublesome antiarrhythmic drugs may be avoided with little additional risk to the patient who has good ventricular function.

Congestive heart failure in CAD is an end-stage of the disease, the result of repeated infarctions that ultimately leave an inadequate amount of normal heart muscle needed to perform the pumping function of the organ. Treatment involves the administration of diuretics to eliminate retained fluid, and **digitalis**, usually in the form of **digoxin**, to improve the heart function. Congestive heart failure from any cause carries with it a dismal prognosis, worse than that of many cancers. Studies show that patients with symptoms of severe heart failure, even when they are at rest, have a one-year mortality rate approaching 50 percent. But heart failure sufferers have some reason to hope these days. Studies of **vasodilators**—drugs that increase the diameter of the blood vessels—have begun to show some promise. Mortality rates from heart failure may decrease in the near future.

CORONARY BYPASS SURGERY AND BALLOON ANGIOPLASTY

Coronary bypass—the surgical creation of vascular conduits from the aorta to beyond the coronary obstructions to restore normal blood flow to the heart muscle—has been the mainstay of invasive heart therapy for over a decade. More recently, another option has appeared for those patients in whom medical therapy seems to be inadequate: coronary angioplasty.

Each procedure, based upon the anatomy of the individual's coronary circulation, his symptoms, and the goals desired by the patient in consultation with his doctor, has its place in cardiac treatment.

Coronary Bypass Surgery

Bypass surgery is performed for two reasons. One reason is to prolong life. The other, almost as compelling, is to improve the quality of life in those people who lead a severely diminished existence because of heart disease.

In order to benefit those patients who, in terms of survival, stand to gain the most from the surgery, a number of cooperative prospective studies have been done comparing the results of medical and surgical intervention. These studies have involved many hospitals and investigators, and many thousands of coronary patients all over the world. To deal with such massive amounts of data and make statistical sense out of it so that broad recommendations for management could be made, it has been necessary to divide patients into categories, albeit somewhat arbitrarily.

Patients have been divided into those with one-, two-, or three-vessel disease, referring to the right and left anterior descending, and left circumflex arteries or one of their major branches. Significant obstruction of the coronary arteries, as determined by angiography, is defined as either a 50- or 70-percent obstruction, depending on the artery or study involved. In any artery, the closer an obstruction is to its origin (proximal obstruction) the more heart muscle will be at risk should it close off, because all the arterial branches arising beyond it will also be deprived of blood flow. Some researchers have attempted to analyze patients with obstructions near, farther, and farthest away from the origins of the left anterior descending artery, since myocardial infarctions involving this vessel tend to be more severe than those involving either the right coronary artery or left circumflex artery.

Given the variability of coronary anatomy in man, and the equal variability of the patterns of coronary atherosclerosis, it is understandable how, even among the experts, differences of opinion may arise with any given patient. Nevertheless, a few findings are worth noting. Obstruction of the left main coronary artery is universally accepted as ominous, with mortality within one year reaching as high as 15 or 20 percent. Surgery is almost always recommended in such cases. At the other end of the scale, a single diseased vessel results in only a 1- to 3-percent annual mortality rate over a five-year period among patients treated medically; surgery offers no improvement in survival. In fact, surgery is rarely recommended for these patients unless their severe symptoms continue despite a regimen of comprehensive medical therapy.

Almost every combination of coronary vessel disease between these extremes is subject to debate, although research has begun to distinguish other groups of patients whose lives may be prolonged by surgery. In particular, regardless of coronary anatomy, the state of the left ventricle's function is an independent predictor of survival. The normal ventricle ejects about half of its blood or slightly more with each beat—expressed as an ejection fraction of 50 percent or greater. A moderately impaired left ventricle ejects only 35 to 49 percent of its contents; a severely impaired ventricle has an ejection fraction of less than 35 percent. Survival data show that patients with three diseased vessels and only a moderate reduction in ejection fraction will benefit from surgery. This may also hold true among certain patients with only two-vessel disease.

The decision to operate in CAD patients would be easier if the coronary bypass operation permanently cured people. But it does not. Much of the surgery involves obtaining strips of vein from the legs and using these to construct conduits from the aorta to a point beyond the obstruction. Unfortunately, any bypassed arteries that may still have had small openings tend to close off rather quickly after surgery. Of greater significance, the veins themselves begin to close off years after bypass surgery, putting the patient back at square one.

Besides the leg veins, bypass is performed using one of the two internal mammary arteries that arise from the aorta and run down each side of the breastbone. The surgeon detaches these vessels from their normal moorings and inserts their ends beyond the obstructions in the coronary arteries. Although they are narrower than the leg veins used for bypass, and the amount of blood that can pass through them is therefore somewhat smaller, mammary arteries are much less susceptible to post-surgery closure. Coronary arteriograms reveal that over 90 percent of these arteries remain open ten years after the original surgery. As a result, one or both of the arteries are usually now used in modern bypass surgery.

Coronary Angioplasty

During the late 1970s, surgeons demonstrated that a catheter fitted with a small balloon could be passed via the ordinary heart-catheterization route to a partially obstructed coronary artery. By expanding the balloon, the constricted point could be dilated. At first cardiologists recommended that this should only be done when single obstructions of limited length were present. As the technique of angioplasty advanced, with improved catheter designs and the growing experience of its practitioners, multiple obstructions in multiple vessels were gradually added to the list of lesions considered suitable for this type of treatment.

The advantages of coronary angioplasty are obvious. In contrast to bypass surgery, the procedure requires no general anesthetic, no chest-splitting incision, and no prolonged postoperative recuperation period. In patients with clear-cut indications for invasive treatment to open up their coronaries, but with other medical problems that make them unacceptable risks for major surgery, angioplasty offers an alternative. In those for whom the need for major bypass surgery is open to question, angioplasty represents a compromise. In patients who have previously had bypass surgery and in whom the veins used for bypass have become obstructed, the balloon catheter can be used to open them up. As a result of all these considerations, probably thousands of angioplasties are now being performed daily throughout the United States.

What are the disadvantages? Not all balloon angioplasties are successful. In some cases the cardiologist may not succeed in relieving the obstruction. There are also potential complications. Data indicate that even at the most experienced medical centers, a myocardial infarction may result from the procedure in about 4 percent of attempts, and the need to rush the patient to emergency bypass surgery occurs in about 3 to 4 percent of cases.

Finally, as early as three to four months following an angioplasty, in about 30 percent of cases, the opened arteries begin to reclose. It is believed that in these cases the balloon has traumatized the inner lining of the coronary artery, thereby stimulating the proliferation of new cells and leading once again to obstruction. Anticoagulants and other drugs are now being used to prevent this problem, but the ultimate success of these therapies is yet to be determined.

Other options to bypass surgery are being explored: **stents** (somewhat rigid cagelike structures that hold the arterial walls open); **lasers**; and **atherectomy**, the removal of coronary obstructions with shaving devices or burrs mounted on catheters. To date, however, none of these semiexperimental approaches has demonstrated significant advantages over balloon angioplasty.

The bitter lesson is that none of the medical and surgical treatments that have been developed for the treatment of coronary artery disease, no matter how advanced and impressive, is as effective as holding back the development of the disease in the first place through preventive health measures practiced by the patient himself.

OTHER TYPES
OF HEART DISEASE

Although CAD is the predominant type of heart disease that confronts the American male, it is not the only one. Disease of the heart valves, **cardiomyopathy** (see below), and disease of the pericardium make up a smaller but not insignificant group of problems that may arise.

Valvular Heart Disease

A heart valve may malfunction in one of two ways: It may not be able to open completely, a condition called **valvular stenosis**, or it may not be able to shut completely, a condition known as **valvular insufficiency** or **regurgitation**. In the past, valvular damage from rheumatic fever and its subsequent heart disease constituted the major problem in this area for Americans. Although still common in the Third World, rheumatic heart disease has become relatively rare in the United States.

Perhaps the most common valvular disorder found today in this country is **mitral valve prolapse**, a bulging of the mitral valve into the left atrium as it closes following each ventricular contraction. Mitral prolapse may occur as part of other heart disease, but more often it is an isolated condition. In many people, especially young women, in whom mitral valve prolapse is relatively common, it simply represents a variant of normal anatomy and has no effect on life expectancy, despite some troubling symptoms that may accompany it.

A more severe and fortunately much less common form of mitral prolapse can result in a leak in the valve, which may eventually require surgery to install an artificial valve. Prolapsing valves that leak (or regurgitate) are more subject to infections. To help prevent such infections, those with mitral valve regurgitation require antibiotics before or after any procedure— dental extractions, for instance—that risks introducing or releasing bacteria into the bloodstream.

Even with mild prolapse, the symptoms can be troublesome. They include palpitations, chest pain, fatigue, and dizziness. They can often be controlled with medication and assurance to the patient of the benign nature of prolapse in general.

Among older people, narrowing of the aortic valve (**aortic stenosis**), often with significant calcification, is a common problem (see chapter 8). Intravenous drug abusers are especially prone to develop infections on their valves, a condition called **endocarditis**, because of their use of unsterile needles. The infections may lead to destruction of valve tissue itself. The resulting leaks, if severe, may require open-heart surgery to replace the valve.

For all patients with diseased valves, artificial heart valves represent a major advance. These devices may be mechanical, utilizing a ball-in-cage design or tilted-disc mechanism, or constructed of biological material to mimic the normal heart structures more closely.

Although valve replacement is a lifesaving procedure and has helped many patients to lead nearly normal lives, all replacements present certain problems of their own. With current valve surgery, sutures can tear loose from the heart tissue to which the valve is attached. Blood clots can form on the artificial valves and prevent them from either opening or closing properly. Such clots may break off and travel to vital organs such as the brain, or into the coronary arteries, cutting off blood supply to these critical organs, with disastrous consequences. Artificial valves are also susceptible to infections that usually prove intractable despite antibiotics, requiring another replacement to eradicate them. To avoid many of these complications, surgeons have attempted to adapt valves taken from pigs for use in humans, but these often calcify or fracture after a few years, and are now limited to use only in very elderly people.

Patients with valve problems caused by coronary heart disease present a somewhat different problem. In these patients the destruction of the heart muscle leads to widening and distortion of the ring of tissue into which the mitral valve cusps insert. Mitral leaking in such cases does not result from valve destruction, but rather from widening of the mitral ring. An artificial ring can be implanted in the region of the anatomical ring to reduce the opening to its original size and allow the cusps to close properly once again. Surgeons often perform this procedure in association with coronary bypass surgery in patients in whom this problem has accompanied the advance of their coronary disease.

Cardiomyopathies

This term refers to diseases that damage the heart muscle directly, rather than as the end result of another process. Cardiomyopathies commonly fall into two major categories: **dilated** and **hypertrophic**. In dilated cardiomyopathy, the heart chambers, weakened by the disease process, expand in size, and congestive heart failure ultimately results. In hypertrophic cardiomyopathy, the disease causes the ventricular walls to thicken.

Excessive chronic alcohol ingestion is probably the most common cause of dilated cardiomyopathies. Many AIDS patients also suffer from a recently recognized form of the disease.

Hypertrophic cardiomyopathy is rarer than the dilated forms, but one type in particular is important because it is among the most common causes of sudden unexpected death in young men. It goes by several names: **obstructive or nonobstructive hypertrophic cardiomyopathy, idiopathic hypertrophic subaortic stenosis**, and **asymmetric septal hypertrophy**. The disease may be inherited or appear spontaneously; it may have no symptoms and go undiagnosed until a young athlete collapses lifeless on the field and an autopsy reveals the cause.

Various medications are used with some success in patients with either dilated or hypertrophic cardiomyopathies. Surgical removal of part of the thickened heart may produce improvement in the hypertrophic form. When these treatments are unsuccessful for the relatively young patient, heart transplantation now offers the best hope for the future survival with a relatively normal range of activity.

Pericardial Disease

Inflammation of the pericardium, called **pericarditis**, is a relatively common disorder. It may complicate the course of many diseases, for example, patients with chronic kidney failure, tuberculosis, or certain connective-tissue diseases. It also occurs as an independent disease among previously healthy individuals, and in such instances is usually caused by a viral infection. Treatment aims at reducing inflammation and pain with anti-inflammatory medications. Occasionally, doctors must drain fluid collecting in the pericardial sac by using a needle or chest tube.

Peripheral Vascular Disease

Disease of the peripheral blood vessels affects either the arteries or veins. Atherosclerosis, similar to that in the coronary arteries, can affect the arteries in the legs. When artery obstruction becomes severe enough, intermittent leg discomfort ("**claudication**") is the most common symptom. Walking provokes a dull pain or discomfort, and several minutes of rest relieve it. The location of the pain relates to the point of obstruction within the arterial tree. Although pain in the calves is the most common site, one may feel it in the thighs, feet, or buttocks. Treatment involves either surgically bypassing the obstruction in the artery or opening it up with a balloon-type catheter.

Common problems with the veins include **varicose veins, thrombophlebitis**, and **thrombosis**. Again, veins in the legs are predominantly involved. Although unsightly, varicose veins are essentially harmless; when severe, they can be removed surgically. Thrombophlebitis is an inflammation of a vein; it is almost never the result of an infection. **Phlebothrombosis** is the presence of a blood clot in a vein, often as the result of prolonged immobilization such as might occur when a person is confined to a wheelchair or to a bed following surgery. Although typically thrombophlebitis is painful and phlebothrombosis without symptoms, it can be difficult to distinguish between the two; in many cases they probably coexist. Anticoagulation drugs are the primary treatment for both thrombophlebitis and phlebo-thrombosis. Treatment attempts to relieve symptoms and pre-vent continued formation of blood clots, part of which can break off and travel to the lung as a pulmonary embolism. Occasion-ally, such an event proves fatal.

WARNING SYMPTOMS OF HEART DISEASE

Many symptoms considered characteristic of heart disease may actually result from other causes, so it is the task of your phy-sician to distinguish among such symptoms and identify the cause or causes.

Chest Pain

More than any other symptom, chest pain is invariably con-nected with the idea of a heart problem. But most chest pain, even in men at risk for coronary heart disease, is related to minor musculoskeletal ailments rather than heart disease. You may not notice that you have strained or pulled a muscle or tendon in the chest wall or upper arms and shoulders until for no apparent reason, you begin to experience the effects a day or so later as chest pain. Muscle or joint pain, unlike typical cardiac pain, is often tender to the touch and feels worse when you move your arms or shoulders.

Problems within other organ systems can cause chest pain. Hiatal hernias (portions of the stomach displaced into the chest cavity) can mimic chest pain caused by heart problems. "Heart-burn," the regurgitation of acid stomach contents into the esophagus, causes a burning pain in the chest. Other esopha-geal diseases may produce similar discomfort.

Pleurisy, or inflammation of the lung lining, can result in chest pain that is especially aggravated by breathing. A ruptured air sac, certain skin diseases, and pain due to gallbladder disease may all result in chest discomfort that can feel like cardiac pain.

Usually your doctor can make a fairly accurate assessment as to the cause of your distress. Very occasionally, to rule out heart trouble and coronary disease in particular, stress testing with or without a thallium tracer may be required.

Shortness of Breath

Difficulty with breathing that occurs when you exert yourself can be a sign of heart trouble. It can also be a symptom of lung disease, extreme obesity, anemia, or simply poor conditioning. Sudden shortness of breath at night that forces you to sit upright in order to breathe comfortably is more typical of heart disease.

Palpitations

This unpleasant sensation occurs when the heart beats too rapidly or irregularly. People who suffer from palpitations feel as if their hearts "skip" beats. Premature beats, those that occur earlier than expected in the normal cardiac cycle, may arise from the atria, from the ventricles, or from the portion of the heart that separates the upper and lower chambers. These premature beats are called **extrasystoles** and do not necessarily signify heart disease; healthy people often experience these symptoms and may not even be aware of them most of the time.

A premature beat often delays the following normal beat. This leaves the left ventricle filling with blood for a longer-than-usual period of time, so that when the normal beat after the extra-systole occurs, the ventricle ejects an unusually large amount of blood into the arterial system. You feel a "flip-flop," as if your heart were "turning over" in your chest. You might have a cardiac problem or be completely normal, but such sensations are often frightening enough to bring you to your doctor's office for evaluation. Even in people with no heart disease, extrasys-toles can trigger rapid heart rates that are often in the range of 180 beats per minute or more, and require treatment. Rarely, people free of heart disease have excessive or complicated ven-tricular arrhythmias. Such people must bear in mind that although such arrhythmias can be debilitating and should be evaluated, they are not necessarily symptomatic of progressive coronary artery disease.

Fainting and Fatigue

True fainting (or **syncope**) involves a temporary loss of consciousness and should be clearly differentiated from feelings of lightheadedness or dizziness. Very rapid or excessively slow heart rates may result in fainting. Those with severe **aortic stenosis**, a narrowing of the valve between the left ventricle and aorta, as well as those people with cardiomyopathies or mitral valve prolapse, may be subject to fainting or dizziness. The other major group of disorders that can cause fainting involve the central nervous system. Most initial investigations of fainting are directed at pinpointing either cardiac or neurological causes for this complaint.

Fatigue is often present in advanced heart disease, but it is a complaint that accompanies many chronic diseases and is therefore unhelpful as a specific indicator of cardiac disorders. Even among completely healthy people, at the end of a hard or stressful day the feeling of fatigue is more the rule than the exception. Fatigue as an isolated symptom is often not very useful to your physician in making the diagnosis of any physical disorder.

Are You at Risk?

Because of the high rate of heart disease among American men, extensive population studies have been made to determine how men in general might avoid developing the disease. A major aspect of such studies involves risk factors—those risks that are fixed and those that are influenced or modified by one's personal health practices.

Fixed Risk Factors

The tendency to fall prey to a given disease almost always involves a genetic element. Some families show a pattern of

Risk Factors for Coronary Heart Disease

Fixed	Amenable to Change
Heredity	Smoking
Sex	Blood pressure
Age	Lipid levels
Race/nationality	Obesity
Diabetes	Sedentary life-style
	Personality (debatable)

frequent cancers, while others clearly demonstrate that CAD is a frequent cause of illness and death among its members. Of course, if we're lucky enough to avoid every other disease, most of us are going to die eventually from some sort of cardiovascular disease. But what the doctor is looking for as he or she takes a history is a pattern of premature CAD, not deaths among octogenarian forebears. Make sure to tell the doctor of any myocardial infarctions occurring in your close relatives during their thirties or forties, or deaths occurring in their fifties and sixties. Such familial patterns increase suspicion of a genetically linked CAD, even where symptoms are minimal, atypical, or even absent.

Gender is another important factor. The onset of CAD among susceptible males in the prime of life is well recognized. Menstruating women, unless subject to other unusual major risk factors, rarely are affected by CAD. After menopause, women increasingly begin to develop CAD, especially smokers and women with uncontrolled hypertension. In terms of CAD, any significant difference between the sexes tends to disappear by the eighth and ninth decades of life.

There are apparent racial and nationality differences in the prevalence of CAD throughout the world. Historically, it has been high among American men, although lumberjacks in eastern Finland have been shown to have one and a half times as much CAD as we do. The western Finns and the Dutch seem somewhat less prone to the disease than Americans. In the past the Japanese have been found comfortably at the bottom of the scale, but recent studies show an ominous increase in CAD among them. Italians, Greeks, and Yugoslavs occupy a middle position. The reasons for such differences are probably genetic as well as environmental. African Americans, who were once thought to be relatively immune to CAD, are now believed to have, if anything, a higher incidence than their white counterparts.

Finally, patients with diabetes have an increased tendency to develop CAD as well as cardiomyopathy that may complicate the clinical picture.

Modifiable Risk Factors

There are a number of risk factors that you can alter in order to reduce your likelihood of developing CAD. The three major ones that have received the most attention, and are clearly the most effective if controlled, are smoking, blood pressure, and blood lipids.

Smoking. The risk due to cigarette smoking rises substantially as consumption increases. The half-pack-a-day smoker has approximately twice the risk for CAD that a nonsmoker has. For those smoking over a pack a day, the risk is three times as great. Those who quit the habit receive early and significant benefits of reduced coronary risk. Within two years of cessation, the risk of myocardial infarction, angina, or sudden death drops to as low as one-half that of those who continue to smoke. After ten years of abstinence, any increased risk on the basis of previous smoking has been erased, and one British study has found that this reversal may occur as early as five years after giving up the habit. The decrease in CAD among American men in recent years may be due in large part to the decreased amount of cigarette smoking among them.

Cigar and pipe smoking have not been as strongly implicated in CAD as has cigarette smoking. For those smoking fewer than six cigars or ten pipefuls per day, the risk of developing CAD is probably very little increased over that of nonsmokers. But for the cigarette smoker who hopes to decrease his risk by switching to cigars or pipe, it is probably not that simple. The typical cigarette smoker inhales deeply, while most pipe and cigar smokers do not. Studies of cigarette smokers who have switched show that the practice of inhalation persists and probably vitiates any potential benefits that the ex–cigarette smoker might otherwise have obtained.

Hypertension. The benefit of blood-pressure reduction in moderate and severe hypertension is undisputed. Among patients with mild hypertension it has been more difficult to demonstrate an equal benefit, especially among those with minimal diastolic elevations, i.e., between 90 and 95. In treating such patients, the cost in time, expense, and potential side effects of medications must be weighed against the extent of new protection obtained. In particular, isolated systolic hypertension— that is, mildly elevated systolic readings with normal diastolic readings—can pose a difficult treatment decision. Although the condition clearly seems to represent a risk factor, it is frequently present among older people who may tolerate medications poorly, and for whom potential benefits are less apparent. Ongoing trials may eventually clarify this issue.

Cholesterol levels. Cholesterol is a fatty substance or **lipid** that is a natural, necessary part of our bodies. Cholesterol is not detrimental in itself, but excessive amounts of this substance in the bloodstream can promote atherosclerosis and heart disease.

The relationship between elevated blood cholesterol and coronary artery disease has been recognized for decades. Reduction of one's blood cholesterol has been shown to provoke a proportional decrease in the risk of developing CAD. Because total blood cholesterol may not be as accurate a predictor of CAD risk as other lipid analyses of the blood, increasing attention has been paid to these lipids.

Cholesterol does not circulate freely in the blood, but rather in association with certain proteins in spherical particles called **lipoproteins**. The most important are the **low-density lipoproteins (LDL)**, which carry between 60 to 70 percent of total cholesterol, and the **high-density lipoproteins (HDL)**, which carry between 20 to 30 percent of cholesterol. Another group, the

very-low-density lipoproteins (VLDL), consisting mainly of **triglycerides**, carry another 10 to 15 percent of the cholesterol but, unless severely elevated, are not commonly involved in CAD.

High levels of LDL-cholesterol are a major risk factor for atherosclerosis, so LDL is known as the "bad" cholesterol; HDL, on the other hand, is known as the "good" cholesterol because many of the HDL particles are involved in removing cholesterol from the body tissues. In other words, elevated levels of HDL protect rather than harm. Total cholesterol that is somewhat elevated but shown to be caused mainly by a high HDL and a normal LDL level should be no cause for concern.

The table below lists the generally acceptable levels for normal and abnormal amounts of lipids in the bloodstream. Men worried about their cholesterol levels should be aware that there is no sharp cutoff point either above or below a lipid level where they are completely free of risk—the risk grows along with the degree of abnormality. At minor elevations of cholesterol and LDL, the risk for heart disease appears to increase gradually, but beyond certain levels in the "high" category, the risk rises sharply and the need for control becomes greater.

Blood Lipid Levels and Coronary Risk in Men
(in milligrams per deciliter)

	Desirable	Borderline High	High
Total cholesterol	Under 200	200–239	Over 239
LDL	Under 130	130–159	Over 159
HDL	45 or greater	31–44	Under 31

Testing cholesterol levels. In practice, the initial step for finding coronary-prone people involves routine total cholesterol measurement. This test is recommended for all adults 20 years of age or older and, if normal, should be repeated about every five years. The aim is to identify susceptible people *before* coronary disease becomes apparent. CAD has been likened to an iceberg: The sudden appearance of angina, myocardial infarction, or sudden death represents the visible tip of the iceberg; the deposits that have been building up for years in the arteries are the invisible and dangerous part.

If your total cholesterol is elevated and has been confirmed, by repeat measurement to exclude lab error and possible fluctuations, then another blood sample is obtained to establish a lipid profile. This usually consists of total cholesterol, LDL, HDL, triglycerides, and total-cholesterol-to-HDL ratio. The profile gives a clearer picture of your lipid status and helps determine the need for treatment.

A few words of caution on cholesterol testing in general are necessary. Popular interest in blood lipids has, fortunately, led to widespread testing in many health-conscious communities. But testing is sometimes done on such a large scale and in such uncontrolled environments—supermarkets and malls, for example—that quality control may be compromised. Blood samples drawn from sticking a finger rather than from veins may lead to inaccuracies. Errors can occur even at a medical meeting—one doctor attended two booths providing this service and found a 35-milligram difference in finger-stick samples obtained less than an hour apart. Abnormalities or possible inconsistencies revealed under such circumstances should be rechecked by a laboratory known to be reliable. Nevertheless, even in specialized research labs, variation on a single measurement can be about 5 percent. In generally reliable clinical laboratories, variations probably range to 10 percent. Incidentally, if total cholesterol is being determined, you need not ordinarily fast beforehand.

Treatment. The first step in the treatment of elevated blood cholesterol is dietary, and involves reducing the amount of cholesterol you consume. You also will be asked to reduce the total amount of fat you eat, especially saturated fat. Reduction of total calories is advised if your weight is a problem, and an exercise program will be suggested that can reduce both body weight and blood cholesterol.

If the initial dietary approach fails to achieve the desired results, you may need help from your doctor or a nutritionist in instituting a more stringent diet. If, following six to nine months of dietary management, lipid levels are still unacceptable, then various drugs can be prescribed to bring your cholesterol under control, along with a continuing diet and exercise program.

The most widely used drugs for lowering cholesterol are niacin and the so-called bile-acid sequestrants, such as **cholestyramine** (Questran). Both types of medication are effective in reducing both blood cholesterol and coronary risk, but neither is easy to take. Flushing, experienced as a burning sensation and a reddening of the skin that can become intolerable, is a typical side effect of niacin. Constipation and gassiness can result from using cholestyramine. Both types of medication need to be taken several times a day for best results, an inconvenience that often promotes noncompliance.

Lovastatin (Mevacor) is relatively new on the scene, and needs to be taken only once or twice a day. It effectively lowers cholesterol, but whether it also reduces coronary risk remains to be demonstrated. A small number of patients, about 2 percent, develop liver dysfunction from the drug.

Many experts believe that some authorities, such as the National Cholesterol Education Program (NCEP) of the National Institutes of Health, place too much emphasis on cholesterol levels as a precursor of heart disease. They point out, for instance, that benefits of cholesterol reduction have yet to be demonstrated in those with only moderately elevated blood levels.

Canadian health experts have taken a similarly conservative view. While the NCEP calls for testing of all Americans over 20, Canadian medical authorities recommend screening only men over 35 who have other risk factors. Lipid levels at which drug treatment is advised are also higher in Canada than here. Until the final answers are in, decisions about when and how to treat elevated blood cholesterol will depend largely on the joint decisions you make with your physician regarding your personal course of action. Generally, the greater the number of other risk factors you carry—family history of coronary artery disease, diabetes, excess weight, smoking, sedentary life-style, high-stress job or family situation—the greater should be your concern that you do not add whatever additional risk is posed by having high cholesterol levels.

Obesity. Some studies have shown a correlation of increasing weight to the development of CAD, but it is not a dramatic relationship. Although we all desire to have an ideal weight, a 10 to 15 percent excess weight probably does not significantly increase coronary risk. But significant obesity—excess weight approaching 50 to 100 pounds or more—is clearly dangerous.

The distribution of excess poundage is also an important factor. Fat deposits in men (and some women) tend to be in the abdomen and upper body, which carries a much higher risk for the development of heart and cardiovascular disease than excess weight in the hips and thighs.

Sedentary life-style. Regular exercise has many beneficial cardiovascular effects: it lowers the heart rate, increases physical endurance, improves the efficiency of the heart by reducing the amount of oxygen the heart requires for any given level of activity, promotes weight loss, and lowers blood cholesterol. It also contributes to a sense of well-being and self-esteem, as well as improving one's appearance.

To date, no study shows absolutely that regular exercise either prolongs life or reduces the possibility of a myocardial infarction, although survival rates from heart attacks are higher among men who exercise regularly than among more sedentary men.

Personality. It has long been thought that the psychological makeup of the individual is a contributing factor in heart disease. More specifically, certain personality types, designated A and B, have been described as having differing propensities for developing CAD. Dr. Meyer Friedman of San Francisco pioneered and promoted the theory that the Type A male—highly competitive, aggressive, excessively time-conscious—is most likely to suffer a heart attack. Conversely, the Type B individual—more passive or "laid back"—is somehow protected by his easygoing personality against the same fate.

Over the intervening years, much medical controversy has surrounded this theory. Proponents recommend therapy to alter undesirable personality traits in their so-called Type A patients; skeptics wonder how strong the association really is, and if an adult man's basic personality can really be changed. They prefer to put their energies into lowering their patients' cholesterol levels and rates of hypertension, or by stopping their smoking.

   Other factors. The long list of possible minor risk factors for heart disease includes excessive consumption of caffeine, the mineral content of drinking water, and the presence or absence of trace minerals in the diet. Most of these theories are fairly speculative, and none are as important as the major risk factors discussed above.

3

Cancer:
Causes and Treatment

Although heart disease remains the number-one killer of Americans, accounting for about 40 percent of all deaths, the various types of cancer combine to be the second most common cause of death among adult men.

WHAT IS CANCER?

Cancer can be defined as an alteration of certain groups of cells within the body so that the normal controls limiting their growth are removed or disabled. Abnormal cell growths, or neoplasms, vary greatly both in their rate of growth and their tendency to spread locally or to distant sites in the body.

The appearance of these cells under the microscope often indicates their nature and their ability to grow without restraint. Those neoplasms that grow slowly and tend to remain localized have cells that appear relatively mature on microscopic examination. They are more likely to be amenable to cure than are the malignant type, and are therefore termed benign. The cells of rapidly growing neoplasms that tend to spread throughout the body (a process called **metastasis**) appear structurally immature. Such neoplasms are much more likely to be life-threatening, and are termed malignant. When the term *cancer* is used, it refers to these more ominous types of abnormal growths. Occasionally, neoplasms that start off as benign may alter their character and become malignant. An example of this might be a polyp in the colon that progresses into a cancer.

Often the word *cancer* is so distressing to patients that their physicians will instead refer to the presence of a **tumor** (from the Latin for "mass"), especially when the type of cell abnormality is as yet undetermined. Strictly speaking, any mass in the body can be described as a tumor—a swelling or blood clot due to some kind of accident, a palpable gallbladder or urinary bladder, or even a pregnant uterus.

The patient and his family, confronted with the dread possibility of cancer, may easily become confused by the bewildering number of terms used by their doctors to indicate or describe cancers. Some of the more common terms are **carcinoma, sarcoma, leukemia,** and **lymphoma.** Simply put, carcinomas are neoplasms arising from glandular tissue or the cells lining organs (bronchogenic carcinoma is a common form of lung cancer). Sarcomas derive from connective tissues (osteogenic sarcoma is a form of bone cancer). Leukemias are various types of blood cancer, and lymphomas involve cancers of the lymph glands.

Causes of Cancer

A number of factors have been implicated as causes of human cancer. Among these are heredity, certain illnesses, indoor and outdoor pollution, viruses, diet, and obesity.

Heredity. Certain families seem particularly prone to the development of cancers, just as others seem to have a greater propensity for the development of cardiovascular disease. Although some cancers have been identified as having a clear hereditary link, no clearly defined genetic factor has been identified for the majority of common cancers. Nevertheless, for those with strong family histories of deaths or disability due to cancer, a greater concern on their part and that of their physicians for the prevention and early detection of possible cancerous conditions is well advised.

Illnesses. Certain underlying illnesses seem to make some individuals prone to particular types of cancer. For example, patients with ulcerative colitis and some rarer forms of intestinal disease have a high incidence of colon cancer over a period of time. Those with cirrhosis of the liver must be watched carefully for the development of liver cancer. Individuals with certain types of lung disease are at a higher risk of developing lung cancer, although both conditions are frequently connected with cigarette smoking.

Pollution. Cigarette smoking is paramount among environmental causes of cancer. It has been implicated as a major cause of an estimated 30 percent of all cancers.

Exposure to radiation by health-care workers and others also has long been recognized as a factor predisposing an individual to the development of cancer. Those exposed to large amounts of radiation, such as the survivors of Hiroshima, Nagasaki, and Chernobyl, all bear an additional health risk. More recently a much more insidious form of radiation has been recognized as a cancer risk—radon gas. This decay product of radium or uranium was first linked to lung cancer in uranium mine workers. When research on indoor air quality began during the 1970s and 1980s, it was found that in homes lying near to ground sources of this gas, there might be an increased risk of lung cancer. A 1988 report of the Environmental Protection Agency characterized radon as one of the leading contributors to lung cancer in the United States, accounting for as many as 20,000 deaths annually.

A number of chemicals and industrial substances have been recognized as carcinogenic: certain forms of asbestos, vinyl chloride, benzene, diethylstilbestrol, chromium, and nickel, for example.

City dwellers, exposed to a number of industrial wastes, have often been described as more prone to certain internally developing cancers. On the other hand, farmers and seamen, with constant exposure to the sun and wind, are more likely to develop skin cancer.

Viruses. Although well established as a cause of cancer in many animal species, viruses have only recently been implicated strongly in human cancer. The hepatitis B virus seems to predispose to liver cancer. The Epstein-Barr virus has been found to be related to a type of lymphoma among Africans. The papilloma virus may predispose women to cervical cancer, and both sexes to bowel cancer. Finally, the HIV virus, which ultimately results in AIDS, is responsible for an unusually high incidence of a previously rare neoplasm, Kaposi's sarcoma, especially among gay men.

Diet. The role that diet and nutrition play in cancer formation has been constantly examined over the years. Evidence of one sort or another has accumulated only gradually and, despite the difficulty in accumulating such data from large retrospective population studies, it now seems irrefutable. It has been estimated that perhaps 35 percent of cancers in the United States might be diet-related.

For example, vitamin A controls self-differentiation among cells. Studies of Norwegian and Japanese men with higher intakes of vitamin A indicate a significantly lower incidence of lung cancer among these groups when compared with others whose consumption was lower than average. Low intake of vitamin C has been linked to certain gastrointestinal cancers. So-called trace elements, those that are found in our bodies in only the most minute amounts, may play an important role in cancer prevention. Selenium seems critical in this regard. Geographic areas in the United States with deficiencies of selenium in the soil seem to have cancer rates higher than those locations with higher levels. Furthermore, patients with cancer have been found to have lower selenium levels than normal.

Dr. Denis Burkitt first called attention to the role of dietary fiber in the prevention of cancer when he pointed out that Africans with high-fiber diets had bulkier stools and less colon cancer than white people living in the same areas but lacking high fiber content in their diet. Subsequent studies in Norway, Greece, and the United States have tended to confirm this finding. However, the effects of a high-fiber diet are more complicated than that; those who consume a high level of fiber tend to eat less of other foods, especially fats, thus reducing the level of cholesterol in their blood. A continuing Harvard study involving a large group of nurses over a period of years reveals that a higher incidence of colon cancer occurs in those who eat large amounts of red meat, which is high in animal fats.

An increasing amount of epidemiological data implicates a poor diet in the formation of certain cancers. The following dietary guidelines are now accepted as conferring possible protection from cancer.

Dietary Guidelines

- Eat a balanced diet that includes all the required nutrients and vitamins.
- Eat red meat only once or twice a week; consume more fish and poultry.
- Take alcohol only in moderation—one or two drinks a day.
- Increase the amount of fiber in your diet.

INCIDENCE OF CANCER IN AMERICAN MEN

The relative role of different cancers that occur in American men may be looked at in two equally valid and important ways. First, what is the relative incidence of the various cancers? Second, which cancers are the major causes of death? For example, although prostate cancer is more common than lung cancer, treatment of prostate cancer is usually more effective. Therefore, deaths from lung cancer constitute a higher percentage of total deaths from cancer. The following table is adapted from National Cancer Institute statistics for 1990.

To interpret this data properly, some additional information is necessary. First, eliminated from this tabulation are all the common skin cancers, which account for over 500,000 cancers per year (see chapter 7).

Although prostate cancer has edged out lung cancer as the most common of male cancers in this country, lung cancer still retains its prominent position as the number-one cancer killer among American men. Furthermore, the above table represents the findings in *all* American men, but the data are dominated by the cancer picture among older men, where the incidence is the highest. Among younger men—those under the age of 35—leukemia and lymphoma constitute the major death threats. Brain, bone, and testicular cancers are also more common in young men than in the male population as a whole.

Estimates of Cancer Incidence and Mortality Among American Men of All Ages (1990)

Type of Cancer	Incidence (%)	Mortality (%)
Prostate	21	11
Lung	20	35
Colon/rectum	14	11
Urinary	10	5
Leukemia/lymphoma	8	9
Oral	4	2
Pancreas	3	5
Skin melanoma	3	2
Others	17	20
	100%	100%

Lung Cancer

As indicated above, lung cancer remains the most common cause of cancer death among American men, with about 90 percent of these cancers occurring among cigarette smokers. Looked at another way, men who are cigarette smokers have a tenfold higher incidence of lung cancer than do nonsmokers. The risk of lung cancer among cigarette smokers rises in direct relation to the number of cigarettes smoked within a given time period multiplied by the length of that period. This is usually expressed by researchers as "pack years."

Lung cancer usually makes its first appearance in the middle years. The incidence is 5.4 per 100,000 of population between the ages of 35 and 39. This rises to 21.6 per 100,000 between 40 and 44; then 51 per 100,000 between 45 and 49, doubling in number by age 54, and doubling again to nearly 200 per 100,000 between 55 and 59. The highest incidence, about 450 per 100,000, occurs in men between 70 and 85.

Symptoms. More than 95 percent of individuals with lung cancer show some symptoms when the disease is first discovered. These symptoms vary widely depending on whether they are due to the primary tumor or to its spread. For example, a lung cancer may cause the coughing up of blood. Or a cancer that partially blocks an airway may interfere with the clearing of secretions and predispose the patient to pneumonia. If the pneumonia does not clear up completely after antibiotic treatment, X rays may be taken that reveal the lung cancer. Some may develop coughs or wheezing as a result of partial airway obstruction and irritation. Occasionally the first hint of a lung cancer is paralysis or convulsions that develop as a result of its spread to the brain. Bone pain due to metastases may also be the initial complaint, as may unexplained weight loss or fevers.

Diagnosis. The medical diagnosis of lung cancer in the symptomatic patient is usually not difficult. A chest X ray will often reveal a mass. Tissue diagnosis is essential because it must be established with certainty that it is a neoplasm. Furthermore, the outlook for the patient and the choice of treatment will depend upon the type of cell involved and the extent of its spread.

A piece of tissue can usually be obtained by **fiber-optic bronchoscopy.** In this procedure a flexible tube with a visualizing apparatus within it is advanced to the site of the mass. A cutting instrument called a **biotome,** mounted at the tip, enables the physician to remove a piece of the mass for microscopic preparation. When the mass cannot be reached, bronchial secretions may be obtained and tested for the presence of tumor cells that are often shed into the fluid. If bronchoscopy fails to establish the diagnosis, the doctor may elect to obtain tissue with a **transthoracic needle biopsy,** in which a thin needle is inserted through the chest wall to suck out some cell samples. If the neoplasm has spread to a lymph node that can be felt in the neck or armpit, a surgeon may remove one of these under local anesthesia in order to make the diagnosis.

Treatment. The choice of surgery, irradiation (radiotherapy), chemotherapy, or a combination of these depends upon the type of neoplasm and the extent of its spread. *Staging* is the technical term used by physicians to place patients in various prognostic categories that enable the selection of proper therapy. In addition, the process aids in evaluating the rate of effectiveness of various treatments in large numbers of patients within each group. Anatomical staging progresses from Stage I, when the tumor is small and localized, to Stage IV, when distant metastases have already occurred at the time of a diagnosis.

Surgery alone may work for someone with a Stage I lung cancer, but once distant metastases have occurred, chemotherapy is usually the treatment of choice. Radiotherapy, too, may be used to decrease the size of the tumor mass and relieve certain symptoms created by tumor size. Radiotherapy may also be used following surgery to increase the chances of more complete cancer destruction at the site.

Unfortunately, many cancers tend to recur after initial surgical or other treatment. This is especially true of lung cancer, which often shows up elsewhere, even though no signs of spread may have been apparent at the time of surgery. Because of this unpredictability, doctors treating lung and other types of cancer often speak of "five-year survival rates" rather than cures. Only after a patient has survived his cancer for a prolonged period, with no evidence of recurrence, do physicians tentatively allow the term *cure* to creep into their vocabulary.

For lung cancer such a conservative approach is, unfortunately, too well justified. Ninety percent of the approximately 150,000 Americans who develop lung cancer each year will eventually die from their disease; the overall five-year survival rate for lung cancer is only 13 percent.

Prevention. Because of the bleak outlook for lung cancer victims, previous efforts on the part of health authorities were directed toward earlier detection of the disease in hopes that those lung cancers discovered *before* symptoms had developed might be more likely to be cured with early treatment. In an attempt to uncover such early cases, it was once recommended that annual chest X rays be performed in those at risk. Although a number of asymptomatic lung cancers were discovered in this way, survival rates were found to be no better for these patients than for those in whom the cancer had been diagnosed *after* symptoms appeared. More-frequent chest X rays (for example, every four months) and/or the obtaining of sputum samples for detection of cancer cells also did not improve the prognosis for those subsequently discovered to have lung cancer.

A particular problem for both doctors and patients, one not usually mentioned in the context of discussions on lung cancer, is the accidental discovery of a **pulmonary nodule.** In most instances, when adult patients undergo an initial medical evaluation or are admitted to the hospital for certain medical or surgical conditions, many of them relatively minor, a chest X ray is taken as part of the diagnostic evaluation. The pulmonary nodule is a density or "shadow" on the X-ray film, usually less than two inches in diameter and often round or coin-shaped in appearance. The great fear, when one of these is found, is that an unsuspected lung cancer has been uncovered. Although some surgical studies have revealed that up to one-third of these do represent lung cancers, most (54 percent) are due to old, healed lung infections. Rarely (4 percent) do they represent other types of neoplasms that need surgical excision. Diagnostic studies, such as those described above, are essential to distinguish among these possibilities, with the chances of a successful resolution of the problem favoring the nonsmoker.

What can you do as an individual to escape the fate of the vast majority of lung cancer victims? The most important contribution you can make to your own health in this regard is never to take up the habit of smoking, or, if you already smoke, to resolve to quit. If one has been a cigarette smoker for a number of years, will it do any good to stop at some later point? Lung tissue destruction and scarring as a result of cigarette smoke inhalation cannot be reversed by stopping smoking, although no further damage will result. As for escaping the risks of lung cancer, the results of kicking the cigarette habit may not be as impressive in terms of reducing risk as they are for coronary heart disease, but they are real. After a period of 10 to 15 years, the risk of lung cancer in an ex-smoker is no greater than in those who have never smoked at all. Although this seems a long time to wait, one should consider that the incidence of lung cancer is greatest in the later decades of a man's life. If you quit at the age of 35 or 40 or even later, the benefits are still quite real in terms of your reduced risk well before your retirement years.

The importance of the elimination of needless radiation exposure must also be emphasized.

Colon and Rectal Cancer

After lung cancer, colorectal cancer represents the most common cause of cancer death among American men. In contrast to lung cancer, early recognition and treatment of cancers of the lower gastrointestinal tract offer real chances of better long-term survival and even cure.

Certain higher-risk groups, those in whom more careful observation is warranted, have been identified. **Familial polyposis** is a hereditary disease with a high incidence of colon cancer. Patients with long-standing ulcerative colitis also are at a high risk of colon cancer. Another major group who require closer watching than the general population are individuals with ordinary polyps of the large bowel. It is currently believed that most colon cancers arise from benign polyps that later turn malignant. Finally, those with close family relatives such as fathers or mothers ("first-degree relatives") who have had colon cancer are at higher risk, as are those who have been previously treated for this type of cancer.

Symptoms. The symptoms of colorectal cancer depend upon the location of the neoplasm (see Figure 3.1). Cancerous lesions located in the right or ascending colon typically result in symptoms related to blood loss and anemia: weakness, pallor, and dizziness. The stool may show streaks of red blood, or, less often, a tarry appearance.

Those neoplasms located in the descending colon, the sigmoid colon, and the rectum are more likely to result in symptoms related to obstruction: difficulty in passing stool, lower abdominal pain, the feeling of incomplete evacuation following defecation, and changes in bowel habits. The appearance of the stool may also change, its narrowed shape reflecting a partial obstruction near the termination of the colon or rectum.

Two-thirds of all colorectal cancers occur in the sigmoid colon or rectum; 50 percent are in the rectum and can be felt by the

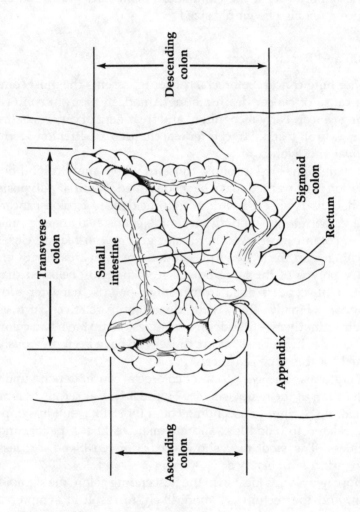

Figure 3.1 The colon or large intestine

examining physician's finger. As with most adult cancers, they tend to occur in the middle and later decades of life, with the first significant appearance in patients above the age of 40. Two-thirds of all colorectal cancers occur in individuals over 50 years of age.

Diagnosis. If the colorectal cancer, symptomatic or not, can be located by a rectal examination, diagnosis is made easy. Where there are symptoms or changes in stool or bowel habits, but no cancer is found on digital examination, the examining physician uses an endoscope, a flexible tube with optical and biopsy attachments, that is passed via the rectum to explore the colon. Polyps incidentally discovered in this way can be removed and sent for microscopic examination to determine whether any have turned malignant. In some patients, a barium enema may be helpful.

CT scanning is also used on occasion in the identification of these neoplasms. Rarely, surgical exploration may be needed when it cannot otherwise be determined whether a particular abnormality is related to cancer.

Treatment. Surgery plays a major role in the treatment of colorectal cancer. Removal of localized tumors, along with adjacent sections of colon to assure completeness of the procedure, can result in a complete cure. Radiation and chemotherapy may be employed after surgery, depending upon the extent and location of the tumor.

In a typical sample of 100 patients discovered to have colorectal cancer, the survival rate in five years will be 27 percent, over twice that for lung cancer. In 25 percent of this entire group, no evidence of persistent or recurrent tumor growth will be evident. Early, localized lesions are especially amenable to successful treatment, with a 10-year survival rate as high as 74 percent.

In terms of effective therapy, colorectal cancer seems to be the one major exception to the bleak outlook for most adult cancers. The mortality for other major cancers—lung, prostate, and breast—has not changed appreciably since 1950. Colorectal cancer mortality, on the other hand, has fallen slightly, although this change has been more pronounced in women than men. Although some experts think this may be an expression of the natural progression of the disease among the population in general, others attribute the improved prospects for survival to earlier recognition and treatment.

Prevention. In 1989 the United States Preventive Services Task Force published screening procedures for a number of cancers. Three types of screening procedure were outlined for colorectal cancer detection: **digital rectal examination, testing for occult (hidden) blood in the stool,** and **sigmoidoscopy.**

A rectal examination is considered an essential part of any complete physical examination. Many colorectal cancers can be discovered in this way and every man over 40 years of age should insist upon such an examination when he undergoes any general physical examination.

When sufficient amounts of blood are shed within the gastrointestinal tract, the stool may be obviously discolored. Smaller amounts of blood in the stool may not alter its normal appearance, and special tests may be required for its detection. Several of these tests have been in use for a number of years. With the emphasis on early colon cancer detection, they have become available from local cancer-prevention organizations, and are even commercially available at drugstores and shopping centers. Such devices should be viewed as part of the diagnostic process, but not as definitive tests. They are subject to false-positive results (resulting from presence of blood or other substances, but not from a neoplasm) or false-negative results (in which no blood is detected despite the presence of colorectal cancer).

Certain precautions must be observed to minimize the possibility of misleading results. For example, it is usually recommended that the test be performed on three or more days. Since ingested meat contains blood that may be detected by such testing, it should be eliminated from the diet for a day or two prior to testing. Ingested iron supplements, or vitamin combinations that contain iron, may also result in false positives. Aspirin is a well-recognized irritant of the stomach lining and may also cause a small amount of bleeding, which can confuse the results. Less appreciated is the propensity for the newer painkilling anti-inflammatory agents, now available without prescription, that may have the same effect. Forms of **ibuprofen** (Advil and Nuprin) are potential offenders. False-negative results may occur if the patient is ingesting large amounts of vitamin C, if insufficient blood is being shed by the neoplasm at the time the sample is taken, if the chemical in the testing preparation for some reason is inactive, or if a positive result is not recognized as such by the person evaluating the color-coded result.

Sigmoidoscopy involves the passage of a flexible **endoscope,** basically similar in design to the bronchoscope (see page 84), into the rectum as far as the sigmoid. Although a somewhat uncomfortable procedure, a number of experts feel it is advisable as a routine screening device for possible cancers in older individuals.

In the final analysis, it would seem prudent for men above the age of 40 to undergo at least an annual physical examination with stool testing for possible signs of occult blood. The patient should seek a second opinion if any questions arise about interpretation of the results.

Cancer of the Prostate

Owing to improved reporting and detection, prostate cancer displaced lung cancer in 1990 as the most frequent important neoplasm occurring among American men. It ranks third, after lung and colorectal cancer, as the most common cause of cancer death in men. It is a disease of older men, the incidence rising rapidly between the ages of 50 and 75. For reasons that are not yet clear, the incidence and mortality among blacks is considerably higher than among the white male population.

A number of factors—genetic, hormonal, venereal, and environmental—have been suggested as contributing to the formation of this cancer, but except for the usual cancer-prevention measures, no specific behavioral or dietary factors seem to be involved.

Symptoms. Signs and symptoms of prostate cancer vary greatly. A physician feeling the prostate as part of a routine rectal examination may feel a hard nodule on the surface of the gland. This is often the first clue that prostate cancer is present. An inability to empty the bladder, caused by a urinary-tract obstruction, may be the first sign of the disease for an individual. In fact, this may be the first symptom in as many as 25 percent of those found to have prostate cancer, when cells are removed from the obstructing tissue and then examined microscopically. Bleeding into the urine is unusual with prostate cancer unless obstruction or infection is present.

At times the initial symptoms of prostate cancer are quite different from what one might otherwise expect. "Arthritis" in the spine or elsewhere may really mean that cancer cells from the prostate have metastasized to the bone, the most common area of spread from these neoplasms. At the time of initial diagnosis of prostate cancer, spread to the bones will already have occurred in between 10 to 20 percent of men so affected. Weight loss, unexplained anemia, and generalized weakness may also be factors leading to the diagnosis.

Diagnosis. Simple palpation of the prostate gland as part of the rectal examination remains the most effective means of early diagnosis. This will reveal the presence of the disease in about 70 percent of those who develop this cancer. In the presence of a suspicious nodule, a **needle biopsy** of the gland is mandatory to establish the diagnosis. This can usually be accomplished with a high degree of accuracy by a competent urologist. In association with this, a number of other tests, including radiology of the bone and certain blood tests, are usually performed to determine the extent of the tumor and the best means of managing it.

Treatment. As with lung and colorectal cancers, prostate cancer is treated according to cell type and the extent of spread in the body. The most minimal disease is that found by chance as part of the treatment for benign prostatic hypertrophy. The slow growth of most prostatic neoplasms, and the fact that they are often found in men of advanced age, means that often no specific treatment is indicated. Such patients often have life expectancies no different from men of similar age without prostatic cancer. In fact, among elderly men with prostatic cancer, more than half will die of other causes.

For larger prostate cancers still limited to the gland itself, **radical prostatectomy** (surgical removal of the gland) can be performed. Another option is radiotherapy, performed either by implantation of radioactive "seeds" or by external radiation. Because in up to one-third of those men found to have cancer of the prostate, the disease has already spread to the bone at the time of diagnosis, another type of therapy is standard: **hor-**

monal manipulation. About 80 percent of prostatic cancers are stimulated by male hormones and can be suppressed by their absence. Suppression is accomplished by the removal of the testes or by the administration of female hormones or newer drugs that either stop the production of male hormone or block its action in the body. Although the results of this treatment are often dramatic, they do not last indefinitely. Post-therapy survival among those so treated is about 50 percent at two to three years and 20 percent at five years. When hormonal therapy is found not to be effective, or has ceased to be effective (approximately 20 percent of all those with bone metastases), radiation therapy may help in treating the cancer that has spread to bones. A final option is the use of **chemotherapy.** Chemotherapy may be effective in the long run, but chemotherapeutic agents in general usually have significant side effects. These include nausea, vomiting, hair loss, bone marrow suppression, an increased susceptibility to infection and, depending on the drug used, possible heart-muscle damage.

Given the variety of ways that prostate cancer may appear, and the relatively advanced age of the men in whom it occurs, many difficult decisions may have to be made along the way. Skilled and well-informed specialists will all have some input: urological surgeons, medical cancer specialists (oncologists), and radiologists (radiotherapists). Because such specialists are only human, and are subject to the natural prejudices to which their particular training predisposes them, their sometimes conflicting opinions have to be resolved by referring to the patient's needs and wants, along with the wishes of his family.

At times, decisions are relatively easy to make. A case in point is an elderly man in whom cancer of the prostate is uncovered during an operation for an obstructed prostate. Here the decision to watch and wait is usually noncontroversial. But what of a relatively young man who has a localized cancer in the gland? Is the treatment to be surgery or radiation? A radical prostatectomy offers a 60-percent five-year survival rate, but the operation has its drawbacks. In the past, almost all patients having this operation suffered from impotence, with another 5 to 15 percent afflicted with postoperative urinary incontinence. Today, newer "nerve-sparing" surgical techniques greatly reduce the incidence of these undesirable aftereffects.

Another option is radiation therapy using newer, more powerful machines that can focus "supervoltages" on the diseased area without damaging adjacent structures. Even a cancer that has advanced slightly beyond the capsule of the gland can now be treated; this has resulted in a five-year survival rate for 70 percent of those treated with radiation therapy.

Although hormonal alteration is usually very effective for controlling prostate cancer that has metastasized to bone, the use of certain female-hormone preparations may predispose the patient to blood-clot formation with possible serious complications. Such side effects need to be added to the equation, although the newer male **hormone blockers** offer a safe alternative to this type of therapy. If hormonal therapy is not effective, or no longer suppresses the advance of the disease, is it worthwhile to initiate a regimen of potent chemotherapy, with all its side effects? Only 5 to 20 percent of those so treated will respond, and the response even with "success" lasts only three to six months, with expected survival following initiation of this treatment only about a year.

Until more effective and nontoxic treatment becomes available and the results of continuing trials with new combinations become known, such decisions will depend upon the individual's philosophy of life as much as upon the science of medicine. The input of an informed and intelligent patient should be part of such decision making.

Testicular Cancer

This cancer usually affects young men between the ages of 15 and 35, and at one time the diagnosis of testicular cancer carried with it the high likelihood of certain death within a relatively short time. Currently, however, it is estimated that roughly 90 percent of men who develop the disease can be cured by surgery (the removal of the affected testicle plus regional lymph nodes), radiotherapy, chemotherapy, or combinations of these. Nevertheless, testicular cancer is still the number-one cancer killer among men in their twenties and thirties.

Early detection is important for successful treatment of this disease, and self-examination is the key to its effectiveness. By simply rolling each testicle gently between the fingers at least once a month—preferably after a warm bath or shower, when the scrotal skin is relaxed—you should be able to feel any enlargement or unusual lump or nodule that may be present. If you do find a lump, have it checked by your doctor without delay. The suspected abnormality may or may not be a cancer, but expert assistance is essential to make sure.

Certain risk factors for testicular cancer are now recognized. Undescended testicles, those that have not normally descended from the abdominal cavity into the scrotal sac by the time of birth, is one. Usually some attempt is made, with hormonal treatment or surgery, to correct this in childhood. Such testicles have a 30 to 40 times greater chance of becoming cancerous than do normal testicles.

Men who have had one testicular cancer are several hundred times more likely to develop it—in the remaining testicle—than are men who have never had the disease. When mumps has been complicated by **orchitis** (inflammation of the testicles), there is an increased risk of later cancer. Those with a family history of this disease are at higher risk as well.

As already mentioned, early treatment is often curative, but if chemotherapy or radiotherapy is required in addition to surgery, fertility problems might result. These, coupled with the inevitable psychological problems experienced by young men with their genital organs so affected, have focused attention on the importance of after-treatment of the patient as well as management of the cancer itself.

Bladder Cancer

This is a disease of the elderly, with the peak incidence occurring in the sixties and seventies. However, it is the fifth most common cause of cancer in men in western societies, and its incidence seems to be on the rise.

The most common early sign is blood in the urine. This symptom may or may not be associated with difficulties in passing urine or with feelings of irritation in that area. **Cystoscopy** (see page 114) is the primary means of diagnosis. Small tumors visualized in this way may be treated with **fulguration**, a burning technique done with an instrument mounted on the cystoscope. Multiple small bladder cancers can be treated with various chemotherapeutic agents. For larger bladder cancers that have extended beyond the inner surface of the bladder and invaded the wall, surgery with or without radiation may be required. Chemotherapy used in conjunction with radiation therapy is being explored as an alternative. The success of all therapy is related to the extent of the cancer at the time of its discovery.

Other Gastrointestinal Cancers

For reasons not fully understood, cancer of the stomach in the United States has decreased in frequency significantly over the past few decades. Cancer of the esophagus and pancreas, however, persist as relatively less frequent problems. They are nonetheless important, if only because of the poor outlook for those who do develop these malignancies.

Smoking predisposes men to both of these cancers. Certain types of tobacco use, such as prolonged use of the pipe with the swallowing of saliva, may contribute to the development of esophageal cancer. Heavy use of alcohol also has been implicated. Esophageal cancer should be suspected when difficulty in swallowing develops (usually solid food first, and later liquids). Symptoms of cancer of the pancreas are often insidious. The first manifestations are unexplained weight loss, fever, or nausea preceding the more dramatic development of jaundice due to bile duct obstruction, and abdominal or back pain.

Unfortunately, treatment for both of these cancers is usually unsatisfactory and mainly directed toward the relief of associated symptoms and complications, rather than toward a complete cure.

Leukemias and Lymphomas

Although not as prominent a problem as the big three—lung, colon, and prostate—cancer of the blood and lymph glands still accounts for close to 10 percent of all neoplasms in men. Especially among younger men, in whom lung, colorectal, and prostate cancer are rare, leukemias and lymphomas take on a much higher significance.

As unfortunate as it may be to develop cancer at an early age, the relatively good news is that many of these cancers respond well to treatment, especially among the young. Thanks to improved combinations of chemotherapy, with or without radiotherapy, many cures are now being obtained for these previously fatal diseases.

Cancer Prevention

Since many cancers occurring in the United States today are believed to be related to life-style or environmental factors, American men should take all prudent steps to reduce their individual risks. For example, the latest report from the surgeon general has implicated tobacco use in one out of four cancer deaths. Stopping smoking is a primary requirement if you want a healthy life that extends into old age. A diet high in fats may contribute to the development of cancers of the breast and colon, and other cancers as well. Avoidance of the sun, especially during the peak hours of 11:00 A.M. to 3:00 P.M., would reduce your risk of malignant melanoma and other cancers of the skin.

Finally, American men and their families should heed the seven warning signals of cancer, as outlined by the American Cancer Society:

> Change in bowel or bladder habits
> A sore that does not heal
> Unusual bleeding or discharge
> Thickening or lump in breast or elsewhere
> Indigestion or difficulty in swallowing
> Obvious change in wart or mole
> Nagging cough or hoarseness

Should any of the above symptoms occur, see your doctor without delay.

THE FUTURE OF CANCER RESEARCH

The research community has certainly not been inactive in seeking new information about the mechanisms of cancer and finding new means of preventing or controlling it. Studies of the genetic aspects of cancer are progressing at a rapid rate and telling us much about how cancer develops at the molecular level. It is now clearly established that our own normal cells contain genes that potentially can cause them to become cancerous. About 30 so-called **oncogenes** have been identified in humans, and, with the exception of red blood cells, are present in every cell type in our bodies. The major questions today concern their normal function and what it is that triggers them to provoke the development of cancer.

Certain viruses may bring about such a process. The hepatitis B virus is closely connected with the development of liver cancer; the Epstein-Barr virus is associated with some lymphomas; the papilloma virus may result in the development of genital cancers. Even though the precise mechanism of these associations may not be understood, control of such viral infections with the use of vaccination may result in a decline in these types of cancer.

Recently it has been found that, in addition to the oncogenes, other genes present in our cells can actually block tumor growth. A better understanding of such tumor-suppressing genes, and finding ways to utilize them against cancer cells, promise a future avenue for cancer treatment. As exciting as such developments may be, the curtain has barely started to rise on the first act of this new aspect of cancer research.

On the other hand, immunological approaches to cancer treatment have been brought much closer to the patient's bedside. Newly developed vaccines against cancer cells show promise. Antibodies specifically designed to combat cancers (**monoclonal antibodies**) are undergoing trials. Increasing numbers of patients in whom the conventional therapies have failed are now being recruited to undergo treatment and evaluation of such innovative therapy. Meanwhile, the effort continues to develop better chemotherapeutic agents and better combinations of agents.

Cancer Centers

While many cancer patients continue to fall into the category of those unresponsive to the usual therapeutic approaches, a new and controversial development has occurred within the medical community: the establishment of private, for-profit cancer centers. Here newer, as-yet-unproved treatments can be made available to those who, for one reason or another, cannot become part of public or privately funded research programs, and are willing and able to afford such treatment as private citizens. These centers are often headed by reputable cancer specialists who have departed the cancer establishment to meet what they feel is a need for the cancer patient community. But they have been criticized by some authorities for offering experimental treatment on the basis of ability to pay.

This is an ethical dilemma that has not been resolved, and a decision to enter such a program must be made with caution and with as much professional and family guidance as possible. Such programs are unusually expensive, and the pros and cons of expending financial resources, often at late stages of an almost certainly lethal disease in an elderly patient, must be weighed carefully.

These programs, however, should not be considered in the same category as those that in the past espoused such blatantly fraudulent treatments as Laetrile and Krebiozen. Such truly unethical practices, which unfortunately still exist in abundance, are usually outlawed in this country, although these "treatments" continue to be readily available just beyond our national borders.

4

The Male Genitourinary System

Disorders of the male and female urinary tract and sexual organs are so common that a variety of physicians, regardless of their degree of specialization, are involved in their diagnosis and treatment. Many problems, for example, can be handled by the family practitioner. Internists are also frequently confronted with such disorders, and obstetrician-gynecologists routinely deal with female genitourinary problems. When such conditions are severe or intractable, it is the task of the kidney specialist or nephrologist to address them from the internal-medicine side. Nephrologists frequently work together with urologists, the surgical specialists in this area.

THE URINARY SYSTEM

The male urinary tract consists of the **kidneys, ureters, bladder,** and **urethra** (see figures 4.1 and 4.2). The kidneys are a pair of organs located high in the back part of the abdomen, one on each side of the vertebral column at a level, externally, just about where the lowest ribs originate. Each kidney weighs about five

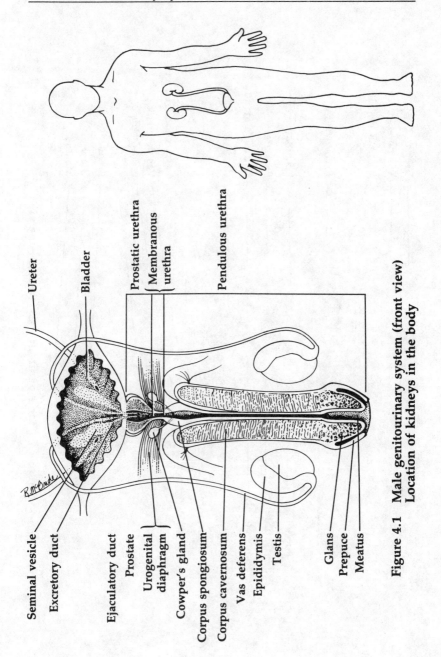

Ureter

Bladder

Prostatic urethra

Membranous urethra

Pendulous urethra

Seminal vesicle

Excretory duct

Ejaculatory duct

Prostate

Urogenital diaphragm

Cowper's gland

Corpus spongiosum

Corpus cavernosum

Vas deferens

Epididymis

Testis

Glans

Prepuce

Meatus

Figure 4.1 Male genitourinary system (front view)
Location of kidneys in the body

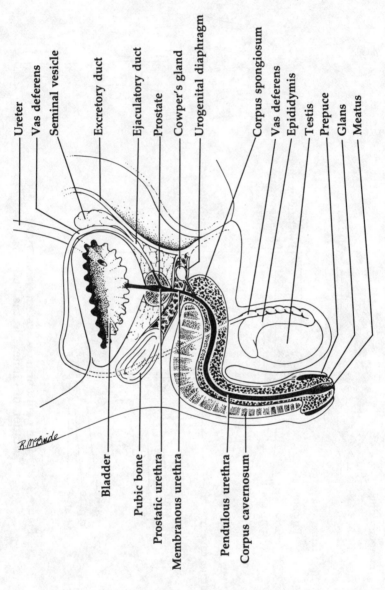

Ureter
Vas deferens
Seminal vesicle
Excretory duct
Ejaculatory duct
Prostate
Cowper's gland
Urogenital diaphragm
Corpus spongiosum
Vas deferens
Epididymis
Testis
Prepuce
Glans
Meatus

Bladder
Pubic bone
Prostatic urethra
Membranous urethra
Pendulous urethra
Corpus cavernosum

R. McBride

Figure 4.2 Male genitourinary system (side view)

or six ounces and measures approximately four inches in length, two inches in breadth, and one inch in thickness. Urine formed in each kidney passes through a long muscular tube, the ureter, to reach the bladder. About a foot in length and a quarter-inch in diameter, the ureters run on either side of the vertebral column to the pelvis, where they insert into the urinary bladder. Bladder size varies depending upon the amount of urine stored, with 17 ounces (or about a pint) constituting the usual full bladder in an adult male.

The lower portion of the bladder narrows, forming the urethra, a seven-to-eight-inch tube through which urine passes during urination (or micturition). The urethra in men is much longer than that in women and is divided into three sections, depending upon the surrounding structures: the **prostatic urethra** passes through the substance of that gland; the **membranous urethra** passes through the urogenital diaphragm, which helps support the prostate and bladder; and, finally, the **cavernous urethra** passes through the penis to the exterior. The urethra serves a dual role in men, in that urine is expelled through it in urination and semen in ejaculation.

Extensive research over the last few decades has shown that the function of the kidneys in maintaining health is a good deal more complicated than just the elimination of waste products from the bloodstream. Although the kidneys perform dozens of metabolic tasks, for the purposes of the present discussion it will suffice to state simply that urine is formed in the kidneys and transported to the urinary bladder via the ureters. Urine is stored in the bladder until, in the act of urination, it is expelled. The kidneys are extremely efficient at their task; even one healthy kidney can perform this function for the entire body. This accounts for the fact that it was single-kidney donation—first between identical twins, later between close relatives, and eventually between strangers with coincidentally close tissue and blood matches—that opened up the whole field of organ transplantation.

Signs and Symptoms of Urinary
Tract Disease

Physicians often categorize urinary tract diseases as "upper" or "lower" urinary tract problems. The former applies to those diseases involving primarily the kidney and its environs, while the latter refers primarily to the bladder and urethra.

Many evidences of urinary tract disease—upper or lower—will be apparent to you simply through observation of changes in your pattern of urination, or changes in the amounts or character of the urine you pass. It is helpful, therefore, to become familiar with some of these changes and the terminology used to describe them.

Nocturia. Nocturia means needing to urinate at night, thus interrupting sleep. Many people have a long-established habit of arising once or twice a night to pass urine, depending upon the amounts of fluid they ingest just prior to retiring. Nocturia implies either an onset of this habit or a progressive aggravation of a previously established pattern. This symptom is commonly associated with various conditions that prevent full bladder evacuation during urination. Nocturia may also signal the presence of a disease having nothing to do with urination itself. For example, it may be an indication of diabetes mellitus, an early sign of heart failure, and even, rarely, an indication of certain types of brain disease.

Frequency. An inability to empty the bladder adequately or irritation in the lower urinary tract (the bladder or urethra) may lead to excessive visits to the bathroom. Closely related to frequency of urination in such disorders are feelings of "urgency," the sensation that one has to urinate soon or incontinence will result. Uncomfortable feelings of fullness in the region of the bladder above the pubic area may also accompany those disorders that result in retained urine.

Polyuria. This term refers to the production of excessive amounts of urine over a 24-hour period. Frequency itself denotes only the number of times daily urination takes place, not the total amount of urine produced. The amounts of urine normally passed over a 24-hour period will, of course, vary widely depending upon how much fluid you drink and lose through perspiration, but it ordinarily does not exceed one and a half to two quarts daily. The most common medical reason for polyuria is diabetes.

Hematuria. This term means blood in the urine. It is usually perceived as the rusty, opaque appearance of the urine itself rather than the presence of frank red blood (pink or red urine). This condition frequently accompanies stones or an inflammatory disease of the lower urinary tract.

Dysuria. This is pain or burning on urination.

Pyuria. This is pus in the urine, which in greater amounts imparts a cloudy color to the urine. Lesser amounts may be detectible only under the microscope.

Urinary retention. This is the failure to evacuate the bladder fully on urination, a frequent accompaniment to obstruction as a result of prostate enlargement among older men.

Urinary incontinence. This is involuntary loss of urine. It is a frequent problem in the elderly male population, for a variety of causes. Other causes are paraplegia resulting from nerve disease or traumatic damage to the spinal cord.

Overflow incontinence. This is manifested by constant dribbling of a distended bladder, usually as a result of urethral narrowing within the prostate, causing large amounts of urine to remain in the bladder. The resulting pressure within the bladder results in small amounts of urine passing out involuntarily.

Self-Observation

Close observation of the color and clarity of your urine can, in itself, be extremely helpful to you in determining whether or not something has gone amiss along the urinary tract. Crystal clear, yellow-colored urine is the norm. Cloudiness may indicate abnormal cellular elements (often pus or white blood cells). An opaque, rusty appearance suggests hematuria. Liver disease or obstruction of the gallbladder ducts results in bilirubin backing up into the bloodstream, causing the yellowing of skin and eyes known as jaundice. When bilirubin is excreted in the urine, it darkens the color to a deep orange or brownish hue, often described as tea-colored.

Fever is a general sign of many illnesses. Where disease of the urinary tract is suspected, however, it may help to distinguish between upper urinary tract infections of the kidney, where fever is often present, and lower urinary tract infections, where it is usually absent, or at least not severe if present. The incidence of kidney infections in men is relatively low when compared to that in women, who, because of changes induced by pregnancy and basic differences in anatomy, have a much higher incidence. When upper urinary tract infections do occur in men, they may be a sign of obstruction lower down, and should lead to a medical investigation of this possibility.

Common Urinary Tract Problems

Genitourinary difficulties, while not as common in men as in women, nevertheless occur often enough to warrant your attention. Older men especially may be predisposed to infections in this area because an enlarged prostate does not allow the bladder to empty sufficiently.

Urethritis. Inflammation of the urethra is the most common male urinary tract infection. These infections are almost always sexually transmitted (see chapter 5). When such infections do occur in men, especially more than once, they may be related to an obstruction somewhere in the area, which requires immediate investigation and treatment.

Urinary retention. Normal urination should completely empty the bladder; any retention of urine is considered an abnormal condition. Abnormal voiding may result from nerve damage caused by spinal cord injury or by injuries to the pelvis. More often, however, any inability to void completely is related directly to obstruction along the urinary tract. Obstruction may take two forms: **intrinsic,** when there is blockage within one of the tubelike passages through which urinary flow occurs; or **extrinsic,** owing to external masses pressing on the urethra and closing it off in varying degrees. In men, extrinsic compression is most commonly due to the gradual enlargement of the prostate gland, through which a portion of the urethra must pass.

Benign prostatic hyperplasia (BPH) describes accelerated enlargement of the prostate. Although called benign because it is not cancerous in nature, BPH is of major importance. It is quite common in older men, and is the cause of so much discomfort as it progresses that it requires medical attention. If not treated,

BPH does more harm than simply causing the discomfort and inconvenience associated with urinary retention—overflow incontinence, the need to urinate frequently, and lower abdominal discomfort. The retained urine can provide a medium for infection. Furthermore, the urine, as it moves back up the ureter into the kidney, can, through the constant compression of tissue, cause damage to that organ.

Although most men over 50 have some degree of BPH, not all have it to the degree that they become bothered by its symptoms. Current studies estimate that of all men reaching age 50, perhaps 20 to 25 percent will require some form of prostate surgery (see below) at some point in their lifetimes. There is no effective medical treatment for this disorder except surgery. Up to the present, researchers have not found any specific predisposing factors—such as celibacy, alcohol or drug use, race, heredity—that can identify men at risk for the severe form of this condition. The process of selection seems to be a random one.

Symptoms. It is not difficult to notice when you have BPH. You will experience a growing difficulty in voiding, and when you do urinate, it will be a weak or inconsistent stream. You will also feel that the bladder does not completely empty upon urination. You may notice, too, an inability to stop urinating abruptly, and a noticeable dribbling after voiding. Your urine may be rust-colored, suggesting blood in the urine. The condition may progress to acute urinary retention—the inability to void at all. (This may sometimes be precipitated by use of certain common drugs, especially cold medications containing antihistamines and decongestants.) In such extreme cases, catheterization of the bladder may be required to allow its contents to drain.

If the diagnosis is BPH, the urologist will perform a cystoscopy to uncover the type and degree of obstruction. The results will determine the most appropriate surgical procedure, if one is required. Occasionally an **intravenous pyelogram** (IVP)—the intravenous injection of radiopaque material that helps to outline the kidneys and ureters on X-ray film—may be ordered to assist in evaluating any suspected problem above the level of obstruction. Urologists may also perform special flow studies to confirm and quantify the degree of obstruction and urine retention.

Although several surgical approaches to the problem have been developed over the past decades, in as many as 80 or 90 percent of cases the relatively uncomplicated procedure of choice is a **transurethral resection.** A cutting instrument similar in basic design to the diagnostic cystoscope is passed through the penile urethra up to the level of obstruction, where it removes a section of the obstructing tissue.

If your prostate is especially enlarged, your doctor may advise that all or part of the gland be removed. The procedures used in this operation are called **suprapubic** or **retropubic prostatectomy.** Both operations involve surgical incisions of the lower abdomen above the level of the pubis. In the suprapubic operation, the prostate is approached for removal through the bladder; in the retropubic operation, the bladder is not entered for the removal of the prostate. Do not presume that any case of difficulty in urinating inevitably results in this kind of extensive operation. As indicated above, the relatively minor procedure known as transurethral resection will be the treatment recommended in 80 or 90 percent of BPH cases that require surgery.

Urethral Strictures

Narrowings, or **strictures,** of the urethra may occur in children on a congenital basis. When found in adult men, such strictures have most often been the result of scarring following attacks of gonorrhea. With the liberal use of antibiotics in the treatment of gonorrhea, the disease does not often lead to urethral strictures any longer. Today such damage is usually the result of some trauma to the pelvis or, occasionally, medical intervention, that has caused some adverse occurrence in the urethra.

Symptoms of urethral stricture are similar to those of BPH, with varying degrees of pain on urination. The location and anatomy of the stricture is determined by a **urethrogram,** a set of X rays taken after a contrast dye has been introduced up through the opening of the penis. The most simple approach to the treatment of stricture involves the passage of thin, flexible tubes of gradually increasing caliber, called **sounds,** into the urethra. They stretch the urethra without causing any new trauma in the process, which in itself can result in scarring. This gradual dilation usually requires several months. If the urologist is unable to pass the sounds with ease, or if symptoms continue to recur more frequently than every six months or so, direct surgical intervention may be necessary.

Kidney Stones

Kidney stone disease, or **nephrolithiasis,** is common in the United States, where it accounts for nearly one out of every hundred hospital admissions. Four out of every five patients with kidney stones are men, with a peak incidence between the ages of 20 and 30. An estimated one of every ten men will at some point within their lifetime experience kidney stones.

Occasionally stones are extensions of a recognized systemic disease seated elsewhere in the body. In patients with gout, for example, one in every five so afflicted will form at least one uric acid stone. In a rare genetically acquired disease, **cystinuria,** cystine stones may be found in the kidney. In **hyperparathyroidism,** overactivity of the tiny glands perched on our thyroids, the blood calcium may be abnormally elevated, leading to stone formation in the kidneys. The presence of chronic urinary tract infections also promotes the formation of stones.

Despite the ability to pinpoint these specific causes of kidney stone formation, in many cases no specific cause can be found. Some genetic linkage is thought to render certain individuals more prone than others to develop kidney stones; there does appear to be a familial tendency. Stones are less common in women and African Americans when compared with the incidence in white American males. There also seems to be a geographical aspect; "stone belts" exist in the Southeast, the Northwest, and the arid Southwest. Inadequate water intake, leading to various degrees of dehydration, seems to be a precipitating factor.

Symptoms. Over time a crystal begins to form in the kidney, growing in size until it forms one or more stones large enough to be visible to the naked eye. At some point, one of the stones enters the ureter, initiating an attack of pain so severe that one specialist has described it as "a misery second to none."

The pain is called **renal colic** because it comes in waves resulting from the intermittent contraction of the muscles as the ureter attempts to pass the stone along. As the stone progresses farther down the ureter, the location of the pain moves from the upper abdomen and back in the region of the kidneys, down into the flank and the lower abdomen. When the sufferer urinates, he will often note blood in the urine that results from the hard, rough-surfaced stone as it moves along, irritating the lining of the ureter. In addition to the pain, this rust-colored appearance of the urine alerts both patient and physician to the cause of the severe distress.

Tests and treatment. A urinalysis is performed as the first step. If blood does not seem to be obviously present, a microscopic examination of the urine may detect its presence. The shape of any crystals found in the urine gives a clue as to their composition and the cause of the stone; uric acid crystals suggest gout, crystine crystals indicate cystinuria. X-ray or ultrasound studies are mandatory in order to locate the stone. Since most stones contain calcium, the obstruction may be visible on ordinary X-ray films of the abdomen. More often than not, however, an IVP is performed for more precise localization and to determine the degree of obstruction, if any, caused by the stone.

The initial treatment of renal colic involves adequate relief of pain through the liberal use of narcotics along with adequate hydration, either by mouth or intravenous feeding. Additional fluid intake is necessary to dilute the urine and discourage the formation of additional stones. It will also help cause the stone to pass. The patient may or may not require hospitalization, depending upon a variety of factors.

In most cases, kidney stones are not more than one-eighth to one-quarter inch in diameter, and the vast majority will be passed out in the urine spontaneously—about half within two weeks and 90 percent within three months. Your doctor may ask you to strain your urine or collect it in glass jars so that any stone passed can be retrieved and turned over to a lab for chemical analysis. This may help both in diagnosis and in future management of your disease.

The larger the stone, the more likely it is to become lodged somewhere along the urinary tract between the kidney and bladder. This condition requires active intervention by the urologist. In the past, stones trapped within the kidney, or impacted at the junction of the kidney and ureter or in the upper ureter, often had to be removed by surgery. The introduction of **lith-otripsy** over the past decade has completely revolutionized such treatment. Lithotripsy is a noninvasive technique in which shock waves are passed through the patient's body to break up the stone into smaller fragments that can then be easily expelled in the urine. The patient is placed in a tub of water or placed on a "water cushion" through which a sonic shock wave is sent. Since its introduction in the 1980s, first in Europe and then in the United States, over half a million lithotripsy procedures have been performed successfully. For stones too large to be passed spontaneously, but still under an inch in diameter, lithotripsy is successful in over 70 percent of cases. To date, no significant side effects of lithotripsy have been noted.

A surgical approach still remains the best option for larger stones in the upper urinary tract, although the number of these procedures has been reduced since the introduction of lithotripsy. Removal from below, using cystoscopic guidance, is still the indicated treatment for stones trapped in the lower ureter or bladder.

Tests Involving the Urinary Tract

Routine urinalysis. Overall appearance of the urine is as important to the doctor as to the patient in determining whether or not a urinary tract problem exists. A urine specimen is carefully examined by eye before it is submitted to chemical testing and microscopic examination. As indicated above, rusty-colored urine can indicate bleeding; cloudy urine may be a sign of pus (white cells) or other types of cells in the urine. The presence and amount of glucose and protein in the urine, as determined by chemical analysis, is often helpful. The presence of glucose may be the first indication of previously unsuspected diabetes; protein in the urine may signal kidney disease. Microscopic examination will provide other information: Red blood cells indicate bleeding, and white cells are a sign of infection. Bacteria or other microorganisms may be present. Certain types of crystals may indicate the individual's propensity for particular types of stone formation.

Urine collections are usually timed; early morning is the best time to obtain a concentrated urine, since there has been no intake of liquid overnight. A "midstream specimen" is frequently requested when urine is to be cultured for infecting organisms. Some bacteria typically inhabit the terminal end or tip of the urethra, and washing them out with the first portion of urine and collecting only the middle portion may avoid the false diagnosis of infection in the bladder or other parts of the urinary tract.

Blood testing. Analysis of the blood is often performed in association with tests directed specifically at the urinary tract proper. The white blood cell count is often elevated in kidney infections, but not in lower urinary tract infections, and this can help your doctor distinguish between the two. When severe kidney damage has resulted in the kidneys' inability to clear the blood of waste, the blood levels of **urea** and **creatinine** will rise. Blood testing may also be helpful in evaluating those patients who tend to form kidney stones, including an elevated uric acid level in those with gout, and calcium and phosphorus levels in other causes of stone formation.

X rays. A simple X ray of the abdomen will occasionally assist in the diagnosis of kidney or other urinary tract diseases. Unusually small or large kidneys may be revealed, or a stone in the kidney, ureter, or bladder that appears as a dense white spot. More often, however, X-ray examination of the urinary tract requires special techniques.

To outline the kidneys and demonstrate the size, openness, shape, and course of the ureters, bladder, or urethra, it is necessary to employ some kind of technique involving the injection of contrast dye or radiopaque solutions. These solutions are usually somewhat syrupy in consistency and incorporate iodine-containing compounds that produce densities on X-ray film, thus clearly outlining the structures in which they are contained. Commonly called IVP (for intravenous pyelography), this has proved to be one of the most helpful of such techniques, and is still considered the primary technique for this purpose by kidney specialists and radiologists.

Many if not most patients will experience a feeling of warmth following the injection of the material. Some may have feelings of nausea, perhaps strong enough to induce vomiting. These are minor side effects. What concerns physicians more are possible damage to the kidneys in some patients and severe allergic reactions in others, especially in those with a sensitivity to iodides, the essential element in the contrast media.

The risk of death from IVP injections has been reported in the range of one in 14,000 to one in 75,000, with the latter probably closer to the truth. (Fatal reactions to penicillin are in the one-in-50,000 range for comparison.) Given the serious nature of the urinary tract conditions for which it is ordered, the risk of IVP is considered acceptable, provided the indications for its performance are proper. Patients with an allergic history or previous reactions to contrast media can benefit from premedication with cortisone-type medications and others, which help reduce the risk. Newer contrast media have recently been developed that will not cause the dangerous reactions sometimes provoked by iodine-containing compounds. Although these new media are still quite expensive, wider use may reduce the cost and make their employment more general.

Retrograde pyelography. This is another technique that has a fairly long history, although with the advent of CT scanning it is currently performed less commonly than in the past. With this procedure, occasionally performed in combination with cystoscopy, contrast material is injected up the ureters through tubes snaked via the cystoscope into the orifices of the ureters draining into the bladder. It has been used traditionally in cases where intravenous pyelography was unsuccessful in visualizing all or part of the ureters.

Computed tomography. CT scanning is one of the newest X-ray techniques in medicine. In the little more than a decade that it has been in use, it has revolutionized diagnostic capabilities in many branches of medicine. Performed with or without contrast media, CT provides film representations of actual cross sections of any part of the anatomy. This technique is exceedingly helpful in determining the character of masses within the kidney (e.g., fluid-filled or solid), or in determining whether a mass seen on standard X-ray film in the region of a kidney is actually part of the kidney or is an adjacent structure. The technique is essentially pain-free and has few risks other than those associated with contrast media and the ordinary effects of any radiation exposure to the body.

Radionuclides. These offer a different approach to the diagnosis of kidney disease. Following injection, substances "tagged" with radioactive elements are detected by special counters designed to pick up their specific radioactivity.

Ultrasound. Like CT scanning, ultrasound has profoundly enhanced the ability of physicians to diagnose a variety of diseases. The great advantage of this technique is that it is truly noninvasive—only rarely is it performed with any contrast material—and no X-ray exposure is involved. Despite millions of such examinations that have been performed worldwide, to date no side effects have been found to have resulted from any application of the procedure. Ultrasonography has proved most useful in determining blockage of the ureters (usually due to kidney stones). It is also helpful in evaluating kidney structure and in examining masses, inflammatory conditions, and calcifications. Bladder and prostate abnormalities can also be detected by this technique.

Cystoscopy. The exclusive province of the urologist, cystoscopy or **cystourethroscopy** is used for the evaluation of the urethra and bladder. The procedure involves passing a tube with a light source and flushing solution through the penile urethra and into the bladder. In addition to its diagnostic value, cystoscopy is used to do certain therapeutic procedures (e.g., dilation of narrowed passages, removal of stones), and can be used to perform biopsies.

Cystoscopy can be performed under general or local anesthesia, and in an outpatient setting. The conscious patient might find the procedure slightly uncomfortable, but in skilled hands and with proper medication he should get through the procedure in fine shape, and should expect no further complications. When used for diagnostic purposes the procedure takes about a half hour.

THE MALE GENITAL SYSTEM

The penis, where the terminal portion of the urethra is surrounded by three cylindrical bundles of spongy tissue (the *corpora cavernosa*), is externally the most visible male sexual organ (see figures 4.1 and 4.2). The opening of the penis is called the *meatus* (from the Latin verb *meare*, "to pass"); the head is called the **glans;** the body is called the **shaft;** and the skin covering the glans is called the **prepuce.** Below the penis, within a loose bag of skin called the **scrotum,** are contained the **testes** (or **testicles**), each with a tubelike structure (**epididymis**) leading to a duct called the **vas deferens.** Also part of the sexual apparatus in men are the **seminal vesicles,** the **prostate gland,** and **Cowper's glands**.

Sperm are produced within the testes along with the masculinizing hormone, **testosterone.** Sperm formed within the testis are transported through its tubular network to the epididymis, a coiled tube that, if viewed upon opening the scrotum, appears to be draped like a chignon over the testis, its superior portion or head somewhat thicker than the inferior portion or tail. The sperm mature within the epididymis.

The vas deferens is a continuation of the epididymis, extending from the tail of the latter to a total length of 12 or 13 inches. It transports sperm from the epididymis out of the scrotum, through the **inguinal ring,** located along the fold of the groin where the lower abdomen meets the thigh, and into the pelvis. Here it runs behind the bladder to a point where it joins the **excretory duct** of the seminal vesicle to form the **ejaculatory duct.** During a **vasectomy,** the vasa deferentia are cut and tied off to prevent the sperm from fertilizing the female partner.

The seminal vesicles, right and left, are lobed structures about two inches in length, lying on the back surface of the bladder. They contribute the major part of the total fluid in each ejaculation (the sperm themselves representing only a small fraction of the semen).

An ejaculatory duct formed by its corresponding vas deferens and the excretory duct of its seminal vesicle enters the prostate gland on each side. The ejaculatory ducts are less than an inch in length and quite narrow, less than an eighth of an inch in diameter. Within the prostate, the ejaculatory ducts empty into the prostatic portion of the urethra.

The prostate gland is the source of many male health problems, and the role it plays is still only partly understood. It is a somewhat conical structure consisting of glandular and muscular tissue, and situated beneath the bladder and above the urogenital diaphragm. The normal prostate in young men is no more than an inch and a half in its vertical dimension and two inches across, although it increases in size with age, especially after 50. Because the posterior surface of the prostate can easily be felt through the anterior wall of the rectum by the examining finger of the physician, variations in the size and consistency of the prostate can be discovered and evaluated by rectal examination. Rectal examination is thus an important component of a routine physical examination for men.

The urethra, following its emergence from the prostate, enters the urogenital diaphragm to become the membranous urethra. Within the connective tissue of the urogenital diaphragm are embedded, one on each side, the Cowper's glands. These smooth, rounded bodies, less than a half-inch in diameter, secrete a clear, sticky substance, occasionally visible at the meatus of the penis just prior to ejaculation. They empty separately through their ducts into the urethra, just past the urogenital diaphragm.

Laboratory procedures to help diagnose disorders of the male reproductive system are not as extensive as for other genitourinary disorders. For the most part, diagnosis is limited to examination of the semen and testicular biopsy for suspected cases of organic infertility, and to specific diagnosis of certain infectious ailments. Prostatic massage performed via rectal examination will cause the outflow of prostatic secretions, which can then be microscopically examined and cultured to detect conditions affecting this gland.

Male sexual functioning has two broad components: procreation and what is usually termed adequate performance of the sexual act, or potency. The first depends upon the ability of the man to reproduce in association with a fertile woman. The second function can be broken down into components: the physical and psychological aspects of the sexual act.

Male Infertility

It is estimated that about 15 percent of American couples are affected by infertility. In 30 percent of these the cause resides solely with the male, and in 20 percent both partners contribute to the problem. Thus, in half the cases, some malfunction may be attributed to the male partner.

Infertility is seldom caused by the man's inability to perform sexually; where infertility is found in a couple, it most often exists alongside full male potency.

What, then, are the causes of male infertility? Exposure to certain chemicals in the workplace can result in infertility. Or previous venereal infections may have damaged the reproductive tract in some way. Men with a past history of mumps that resulted in testicular involvement (**orchitis**) can occasionally experience infertility. An underlying genetic or endocrine disorder may exist, and either a geneticist or an endocrinologist may be able to contribute to an accurate diagnosis.

Usually, however, the cause is not obvious, and a urologist will have to analyze the patient's semen to determine the number and appearance of his sperm. Such analysis will yield the approximate number of viable sperm; any other findings (such as abnormal motility of sperm) are of assistance in making the proper assessment. Rarely, a biopsy of the testicles is necessary to help in the evaluation.

No specific cause for the inability to produce adequate numbers of functioning sperm is found in about 25 percent of infertile men. Such cases of infertility are termed "idiopathic." Attempts to treat such cases with a variety of hormonal or other modalities have not produced consistent results. Often, a physician who blindly persists in this frequently unproductive approach can cause increased frustration and anger in his patient. You would be better served by a doctor who, early on, is fully candid about your true prospects for success, so that you and your partner can, if you both so choose, pursue alternative avenues to parenthood, such as adoption, artificial insemination, and so forth.

Other causes. Male infertility has other causes; one is involuntary, the other is not. A **varicocele,** for example, can result in infertility. This is an abnormal dilation of the network of scrotal veins, where they leave the scrotum en route back to the pelvis. The condition will show in about one-third of men appearing in infertility clinics for diagnosis and treatment. The condition is readily apparent as a wormlike collection of veins within the upper part of the scrotum.

Varicoceles have been associated with infertility since antiquity, although the association is not always inevitable. An analysis of semen usually shows an abnormality in some, but not all, of those with the condition. It is not known precisely how the varicocele causes this effect, but the surgical removal of the varicocele will result in improved semen quality in two-thirds of men so treated, with a follow-up pregnancy rate in their partners of approximately 40 percent. Thus, finding a varicocele in the male partner of an infertile couple is cause for optimism.

Vasectomy has become a popular method of permanent birth control for American men over the past few decades. The procedure can be done in the doctor's office, using a local anesthetic. The doctor makes a small incision in the scrotum and cuts the vas deferens, the tube that carries sperm. There may be some resulting soreness, but this lasts only a few days. Because it takes a number of weeks until the sperm stored in the testicles is eliminated, the man or his partner must use some other means of contraception before he is totally sperm-free.

Vasectomies do not affect a man's health or his ability to function sexually. Sometimes a man who has undergone this procedure wants a reconstitution of the vas deferens in order to permit future child-bearing. **Vasovasotomy** is the name given to the surgical procedure used to repair the vas deferens. Currently, most of these operations are performed using an operating microscope. A success rate of 71 percent has been achieved by a pioneering specialist of this procedure, and this remains the standard for the skillful and experienced surgeon. However, success rates are often lower.

Impotence

Impotence, or the failure of the male to achieve an adequate erection for performance of the sexual act, was once considered primarily a psychological problem. Today, however, it is recognized that many physical conditions can result in impotence (see chapter 5).

Ejaculatory Disorders

The culmination of the male sexual act is the delivery of semen to the partner by ejaculation. The most common physical disorder regarding this final phase is **retrograde ejaculation,** in which, instead of issuing from the penis, the semen is directed back into the man's bladder.

Retrograde ejaculation is a possible diagnosis if you experience a "dry" ejaculation, or pass cloudy urine following the sexual act. The cause or causes can include previous trauma to the pelvic area, structural damage as a result of surgical intervention, congenital malformations of the urethra, spinal cord injuries, diabetes, and the use of certain drugs. Finally, there is the inevitable "idiopathic" category, where no specific cause can be identified.

The urologist makes the diagnosis by finding significant numbers of sperm in the bladder urine. The success of therapy will depend on the physician's ability to address and correct the underlying cause.

Another, less common, problem involving ejaculation is ejaculatory failure, in which very little or no ejaculate is produced. Much more common is **premature ejaculation,** a common complaint of a psychological nature, which is discussed in chapter 5.

Testis and Scrotum Disorders

Orchitis. This is an infection of the testes, and is usually related to a more generalized infection. The orchitis that occurs as a residual effect of mumps is of interest to men because of the frequency of this viral disease. Mumps orchitis occurs in about 18 percent of male mumps cases, but is rare when the mumps occur before puberty. About 70 percent of orchitis cases involve only one testis. Treatment during an acute attack is usually limited to pain relief, scrotal support, and bed rest. Subsequent infertility following an attack of mumps orchitis is most likely to occur when both testes have been affected, but the resulting infertility rate is still probably less than 10 percent.

Testicular torsion, or twisting of the testis, is considered a surgical emergency. In addition to the attendant pain, the twisting of the testis can cut off blood supply to the organ and cause permanent damage if surgery is not performed as soon as possible. The main symptom is sudden acute pain in the scrotal area. Torsion occurs most commonly at puberty, between the ages of 12 and 18, the incidence falling off gradually thereafter. The prognosis is good if surgery is performed within four to six hours of the attack.

Swelling or increased size of the testis or its coverings may indicate the presence of a neoplasm or tumor (see chapter 3). Other swellings within the scrotal sac include the varicocele, mentioned previously, and the **hydrocele.** The hydrocele, the most common abnormal scrotal mass, is a collection of fluid within the scrotum between the two layers of membrane surrounding the testis. The formation of a hydrocele may occur secondarily to other testicular conditions, and this possibility should certainly be considered by your physician. Most often, however, if the mass can be tolerated without discomfort, and if it does not seem to be growing, simple periodic medical observation may be all that is called for. If it increases in size to the point that it causes discomfort, surgery can provide relief.

Epididymitis is an acute inflammation of the epididymis. It is most commonly associated with a sexually transmitted disease (see chapter 5).

Disorders of the Penis

Many penile problems are congenital and can be corrected surgically early in childhood. Among adults, penile lesions usually are venereal in nature (see chapter 5). However, there are some rarer causes of penile dysfunction.

Balanitis refers to infections of the end of the penis (the glans) and is almost invariably associated with the overhanging foreskin (prepuce) in uncircumcised males. The role of circumcision, performed shortly after birth, in preventing this and other disorders later in life is a subject of current controversy. Some experts maintain that good personal hygiene will prevent most of the complications related to the uncircumcised penis in adult men. Others continue to recommend circumcision, which is still performed on a majority of newborn American males, although the numbers are declining.

Paraphimosis is a condition occurring in uncircumcised men in which the foreskin becomes retracted behind the glans, begins to swell, and cannot be brought forward. Surgical intervention is required.

Priapism is a rare, painful condition producing a prolonged erection unassociated with any sexual impulses. It may be related to underlying blood disorders or to the effects of certain drugs. A variety of medical and surgical treatments are available for relief.

Prostatitis

An inflammation of the prostate gland, **prostatitis** is a common condition. It may be acute or chronic; it may be bacterial in nature or not; it may be associated with abnormalities of prostatic secretions or not. Four types of prostatitis are currently recognized.

Acute bacterial prostatitis. This condition is accompanied by the sudden onset of fever, chills, lower back pain, and discomfort in the perineum (the area between the anus and the scrotum). The physician makes the diagnosis by feeling a swollen, tender prostate on rectal examination. Massaging the gland will express its secretions from the tip of the penis. The presence of inflammatory cells and bacteria will confirm the diagnosis. Such acute attacks usually respond well to antibiotic treatment.

Chronic bacterial prostatitis. Less dramatic than acute bacterial prostatitis, this is usually associated with recurrent urinary tract infections, and symptoms of the infection may predominate over any prostatic discomfort. The patient's response to antibiotics is also less immediate, and so treatment is more prolonged.

Nonbacterial prostatitis. The most common chronic form of the condition, in this variety no bacterial culprit can be identified on examination and culture of the prostatic secretions. Other microorganisms have been implicated as causes of the condition, but many questions still remain. Clinically, this form of prostatitis resembles the chronic bacterial type and is differentiated only in that no bacteria are found in the prostatic secretions. Antibiotics are of no help in this condition, and so the treatment is symptomatic and supportive. Certain drugs that modify the nervous control of the bladder (**anticholinergics**) may relieve any feelings of urgency and pain. Anti-inflammatory agents such as **indomethacin** (Indocin) and **ibuprofen** (Motrin, Nuprin, Advil) can be helpful. Hot sitz baths may relieve pelvic discomfort.

Prostodynia. This form of prostatitis is also chronic, but here examination of prostatic secretions reveals no evidence of inflammation or infection. It is seen most commonly in men between the ages of 20 and 45, with the predominant symptom being pain or pressure in any one of several regions in the pelvic area (the scrotum, pubis, perineum). These men frequently also have some complaint related to voiding, and special studies of this function usually reveal abnormalities of flow. Treatment is directed to the urinary complaint, with supportive measures for other symptoms associated with the condition.

5

Sexual Health for Men

There are five psychophysiological phases of male sexual response: **appetitive** or **libido** (interest in and desire to have sex); **erection** (transition of the penis from a limp to an erect state); **ejaculation** (the release of semen); **orgasm** (the pleasurable feeling following ejaculation); and **detumescence** (the loss of erection after ejaculation). A period ensues, lasting from several minutes to as long as several hours, during which time further sexual arousal to the point of erection cannot be achieved.

Sexual adequacy in the adult male often has been equated with the frequency with which the cycle of the sexual act can be accomplished and repeated. It is now common knowledge that the sexual athleticism of adolescence is only a phase; that with increasing age and maturity it is the quality rather than the quantity of sex that becomes more important; and that there is a broad spectrum encompassing the normal range of sexual desire and activity for men, and for women as well.

Perhaps the most reliable determinant of whether there is a problem of sexual functioning is the perception by either partner that a problem exists. Concerns about male sexual functioning are focused almost exclusively on impotence, ejaculatory problems, and loss of desire for sex.

SEXUAL DYSFUNCTIONS AND DISORDERS

Impotence

Impotence, defined as the inability to maintain an erection firm enough for sexual intercourse, is one of the most frequently expressed sexually based complaints among men. **Primary impotence,** in which an adequate erection has never been achieved, is rare. **Secondary impotence,** in which one has had previous success and now experiences difficulty, is by far the more common situation. Erectile dysfunction should not be confused with sterility. In the latter, the male performance of the sexual act may be perfectly adequate, but quantities of effective sperm adequate for the purpose of reproduction are not produced.

It is being recognized increasingly that the physical causes of impotence are as important as the psychological causes. Besides actual physical defects or diseases that suppress libido or interfere with erection, factors such as commonly prescribed medications are now looked at for their role in contributing to impotence. Certain types of drugs such as beta blockers, used in the treatment of hypertension, migraine, and tremors, are notorious in this regard. Impotence has been described following use of a popular anti-ulcer drug, **cimetidine** (Tagamet). Psychoactive antidepressant drugs—the tricyclics and the monoamine oxidase inhibitors—have been implicated in sexual malfunction. In truth, at some time or other, almost every commonly used drug has been suspected of such side effects. The general rule is that *any* drug may be involved in *any* untoward side effect in *any* individual.

Those temporarily or chronically incapacitated from any illness may experience a lack of sexual drive or inability to perform. Starvation diets and physical exhaustion may have similar inhibitory effects. Alcohol and certain illicit drugs may reduce inhibitions, but also may adversely affect sexual performance. Family strife, business worries, professional preoccupations, and marital discord, along with more-subtle psychosocial influences, may all follow a man into the bedroom and result in sexual malfunction. The disorder often feeds on itself, with fears about inability to perform exacerbating the problem.

It is important to remember that all men, at one time or another, usually for never-to-be-explained reasons, have experienced or will experience episodes of impotence.

In truth, the need to "perform" weighs heavier on men than on women. A woman, even though unaroused, can physically accommodate her partner and allow him to gratify himself. If she so chooses, she can feign orgasm to add to his pleasure. As for the man, he cannot fake an erection, and when his organ begins to fail him at these critical moments, it may take all the physical and emotional resources of both partners to restore his potency. At times, some professional assistance may be required as well. **Sensate focus exercises,** or touching, popularized by Masters and Johnson and now widely used, are often a component in such therapy. Touching progresses from nonsexual parts of the body to sexual areas, with full sexual functioning as the ultimate goal.

Physical causes of impotence. Penile erection involves a complex interaction of a combination of neurological, vascular, and hormonal factors, as well as a psychological component. All of these combine to result in the engorgement of the penis with blood, which gives it a rigidity adequate for sexual penetration.

The physical reasons for impotence are many. Impotence has been shown to be related to an insufficient supply of blood to the pelvic area containing the penis and associated structures; to nerve damage involved with spinal cord injury; and to certain brain disorders. Abnormalities of the endocrine system can result in inadequate male hormone production and therefore in impotence. More important is the possibility of diabetes mellitus, probably the most frequent single cause of impotence in the United States. At least half of all diabetic men complain of some degree of impotence, believed to be the result of nerve damage from the disease. Although impotence is more common in older diabetics, the complaint may also occur in younger diabetic men and does not seem to be related to the adequacy of their diabetic control with insulin or other oral medications used in the treatment of the disease.

Not to be overlooked as precipitating factors in impotence are alcohol, drugs, and medications. About the first, Shakespeare put it best: "It provokes the desire, but it takes away the performance." The effects of drugs on impotence depend upon the drug taken. Narcotics unquestionably diminish interest as well as ability to perform the sexual act. Stimulants are less clearly implicated. A variety of medications, especially some of those commonly used in treatment of high blood pressure or coronary heart disease, have a well-known propensity for causing sexual dysfunction in some patients. Any man on any new medication who notices a change in sexual performance should immediately ask his physician if any such effects have been reported for the medication he is taking.

Treatment. If no specific remediable cause for the impotence has been identified, and psychological causes have also been ruled out, a variety of medical approaches can be attempted by the physician.

The use of male hormone in cases where no definite endocrine abnormality has been identified is usually fruitless. However, physicians should routinely measure serum testosterone levels in impotent patients; hormonal abnormalities, once thought to be a rare cause of impotence, are now recognized with increasing frequency.

Drugs that cause dilation of the penile blood vessels have also been employed with a variable success rate. But the lack of consistent results with pharmaceutical approaches has led to the development of various prosthetic devices. These devices include penile implants, which can be inflated by the patient prior to engaging in sex. Another approach involves externally applied vacuum-type devices that induce erections by sucking blood into the corpora cavernosa. Finally, direct surgical revascularization of the penis (rebuilding of the penile blood vessels) has also been tried in some cases, with varying degrees of success.

Problems with Ejaculation

Early or premature ejaculation is a common problem among men, compromising the man's ability to sustain coitus long enough to stimulate his sexual partner to climax. An extreme form of this occurs when the man ejaculates even before penetration. More often, it occurs a short time after initiation of coitus. How short a time qualifies as "premature"? This is very subjective and highly variable in interpretation. Perhaps the best definition of a premature ejaculation is one that occurs earlier than either partner desires.

In some cases an early ejaculation presents no problem. If a second erection can be achieved within a reasonable time, a number of men find it much easier to hold off a second ejaculation. To assist men in prolonging time before ejaculation, anesthetic creams have been prescribed, with variable effects. The use of a condom may also decrease penile stimulation and thus prolong the time to ejaculation. Temporary cessation of thrusting may delay ejaculation, although loss of erection can also occur if this is repeated too often. Understanding, experimentation, planning, and patience on the part of both partners are essential in overcoming such difficulties. If these efforts fail, professional counseling may be required.

The opposite of premature ejaculation is failure to ejaculate, or **ejaculatory incompetence.** In the experience of Masters and Johnson, the most common pattern (in two-thirds of patients) is **primary ejaculatory incompetence,** in which men have never been able to ejaculate during intercourse. In the remaining third, the ability to ejaculate during intercourse has been lost. In about 85 percent of such cases, however, masturbatory ejaculation is possible.

Less extreme than ejaculatory incompetence, but far more common, is **retarded ejaculation,** in which the time from initiation of coitus to ejaculation is excessively prolonged. In both conditions, to some extent, this may prove pleasurable to the sexual partner. Among some partners, however, this may develop into a source of resentment. The inability of the man to ejaculate may be interpreted by the partner as a feeling on his part that the partner is either insufficiently attractive or not sexually competent enough to bring him to orgasm. Prolonged thrusting of the male may also result in pain or fatigue in the partner. Sexual counseling, including sensate focus exercises, may help resolve such problems.

Inadequate Sexual Desire

A growing loss of interest in sexual activity in a man who previously experienced a "normal" desire for sex may occasionally result from physical causes, some of which have been enumerated as causes of impotence. Rarely do hormonal deficiencies result in loss of desire. Depression, though, may be accompanied by a decrease in libido. For the most part, the decreasing interest in sex can be ascribed to less severe psychological factors and to a variety of other personal and social situations. Money problems, family tensions, and other types of anxiety-producing discord can lead to a diminishing interest in sex.

How little sexual activity must there be before it constitutes a problem? The range of "normal" sexual activity is wide. Some couples make love nightly or even more frequently; others are satisfied with the act once or twice a month. Most long-term compatible couples realize that there is more to a loving relationship than copulation, and succeed in expressing affection through touch and words as well. Problems do not seem to arise except when an acute imbalance in the need or desire for sexual activity exists between the two parties.

Individual approaches to the resolution of such disparate needs are possible without resort to professional help or even dissolution of the relationship. The more passive partner may agree to the more urgent demands of a mate in order to keep the relationship stable. The more strongly interested party may endure something less than what that individual considers a full complement of sex for the same reason. An apparent loss of interest in sex for a man may be the result of a problem with impotence or premature ejaculation. Rather than face the crisis of imperfect performance repeatedly, avoidance of the act altogether may be his imperfect solution. In the latter case, recourse to sexual therapy would undoubtedly be a preferable choice.

Sexual aversion is to be distinguished from loss of sexual desire; in the former there exists a pathological fear in regard to the sex act, so much so that the possibility of sex can provoke all the physical sensations of phobias (see chapter 6). Sexual aversion may be related to the inculcation in the patient during childhood of negative attitudes about sex. It may also be the consequence of early traumatic sexual experiences such as rape, incest, or problems of gender confusion. All of these problems can be resolved or at least modified by competent sexual therapy.

Sex Therapy

If you decide to seek advice, your first stop should be your personal physician. He or she knows you best and can rule out various physical causes and perhaps discuss with you some relatively simple possible solutions. If the problem proves outside your doctor's area of professional competence, he or she can advise you on how to seek other professional assistance.

Once strictly the province of conventional psychiatry, therapy for sexual malfunction has undergone major changes over the last two or three decades. As pioneered by Masters and Johnson, therapy for both partners of a distressed relationship has become a popular approach to treatment. The aim is rapid diagnosis and intensive treatment of the condition; a two-week period of total commitment is usually required to accomplish these goals. Masters and Johnson report about an 80-percent success rate using their techniques.

Other acceptable approaches to sex therapy involve weekly sessions over a longer period. A pair of therapists need not necessarily be employed to achieve the desired results. In some cases where basic underlying psychological problems are involved, a somewhat prolonged period of psychotherapy may be your best choice. To date, many different techniques have been employed, with acceptable success rates reported by the practitioners and their advocates.

A field so emotionally charged presents an opportunity for all kinds of fraud, misrepresentation, and quackery. Some sex therapists have been guilty of personal participation in sexual acts with their clients, a practice that is clearly an abuse of professional ethics. Others in the field have prescribed "surrogate partners," some of whom may be well trained and serious about their endeavors, while others are not, and consider surrogacy an opportunity to earn easy money.

To avoid potential pitfalls, it is important for you to seek guidance from physicians who are well informed about reliable sources of assistance. If your doctor is unfamiliar with the field, or uninterested in it, you can get help from two professional organizations that have been established for the guidance of those seeking reliable, professional sex therapy: the Society for Sex Therapy and Research, located in New York City; and the American Association of Sex Educators, Counselors and Therapists (AASECT), in Washington, D.C. Most, if not all, responsible and qualified practitioners are registered with one of these organizations.

Never hesitate to ask about the qualifications of any practitioner with whom you are about to entrust your personal well-being. In this area especially, you must have absolute confidence in the competence of the therapist. If you are uneasy with him or her, seek assistance elsewhere.

BIRTH CONTROL

The responsibility for preventing pregnancy has fallen predominantly upon women, especially since the introduction of "the pill." Those who are not using some form of estrogen therapy (the pill) are using diaphragms, spermicidal agents, intrauterine devices (IUDs), or cervical caps or sponges, or have undergone voluntary sterilization.

Statistically, between 60 and 80 pregnancies will occur annually among 100 fertile, sexually active women if no form of birth control is employed. It is against these figures that the effectiveness of any form of contraception is measured. The table below gives the effectiveness rate of the most popular birth-control methods used today. Withdrawal before ejaculation is not indicated here because sperm may find their way into the vagina even before the man senses imminent orgasm and withdraws. The rhythm method, which depends upon calculation of a woman's "safe" periods during the menstrual cycle, is also of questionable value. Intrauterine devices, because

Effectiveness of Birth-Control Methods

Method	Pregnancies per 100 women per year
Combination pill (estrogen plus pro-gesterone)	Less than 1
Diaphragm with spermicide	2–20
Vaginal spermicide—foam	2–29
Vaginal spermicide—jellies or creams	4–36
Condom	3–36
Rhythm method	1–47
Norplant	Less than 1

of past problems, are now used more selectively, and are not popular with the large majority of sexually active women.

A significant number of women today elect voluntary sterilization. This involves cutting or tying the fallopian tubes, through which a mature egg (or ovum) is transported monthly to the uterus, where it can be fertilized by the male's sperm. **Tubal ligation** is the common term used to describe this procedure. Most often a tubelike instrument called a **laparascope** is introduced through a small abdominal surgical incision and the tubes are closed off, using a coagulation or burning technique. Both methods are highly successful in preventing later pregnancies. Bear in mind that restoration of tubal "patency" or openness following a tubal ligation that uses suture material has about a 70-to-80-percent chance of success, but a restoration of coagulated fallopian tubes to patency is considerably more difficult.

Newer methods of female contraception include one in use in France. It is a pill taken *after* intercourse, when possible fertilization may have occurred, and it causes a spontaneous abortion of the fetus. For reasons more political and social than scientific, it has not been introduced into the United States at this time.

The latest innovation in long-term birth control is **Norplant,** a product that has recently received FDA approval for marketing in the United States. A set of tiny tubes containing hormones are inserted under the woman's skin (usually in the arm) by means of a puncture or incision. The tubes can be left in place for up to five years, but can be removed easily by a physician at any time. According to all the most recent studies, Norplant provides almost complete protection—the failure rate is only 1 percent—for a period of five years.

To date, there are no known side effects of Norplant. Approximately 10 percent of women will not be able to use this form of contraception because of menstrual irregularities.

The Role of Men in Preventing Pregnancy

It seems as if the male of the species has little to do in this vital area of sexual relationships. Not so. Although his options may be limited, every man has a responsibility both to himself and to his partner to make sure that some type of prevention is practiced to avoid the chance of an unwanted pregnancy *before* it happens.

To date, there are only two effective methods of contraception that can be used by the man: condoms and sterilization.

Condoms

In the past, most men used condoms mainly for protection against disease and incidentally to prevent pregnancy in their partners. Today condoms have again found favor largely because of the emergence of AIDS and other sexually transmitted diseases (STDs). Combined with the use of spermicides, however, condoms offer a highly reliable form of birth control.

Failure to achieve high levels of protection occurs when the same condom is used more than once, or if the penis is allowed to remain in place too long within the vagina following ejaculation, and semen leaks out. In some instances, when couples regularly using condoms take a chance from time to time and forgo their use, pregnancy is often the result.

Besides protection against pregnancy, condoms have other advantages. With lubricated condoms, penetration is easier and intercourse more comfortable. Then, too, men who have difficulty with premature ejaculation may find that the use of a condom can enable them to control this tendency more effectively.

On the potential downside, some couples complain of a loss of spontaneity when a lovemaking session has to be interrupted for the donning of a contraceptive device. Some men may experience a loss or weakening of the erection in the time the condom is located, unwrapped, and fitted over the penis. Others complain that a condom reduces sensory stimulation of the penile shaft during intercourse, detracting from their enjoyment. It is foolish, however, to hold to the absurd and outdated notion that refusal to wear a condom represents some sort of romantic machismo or sexual bravado.

Vasectomy

A man also has the option of undergoing voluntary sterilization, or vasectomy, which consists of cutting and tying off each of the vasa deferentia, the tubes that transport sperm from the testes to the penis.

A vasectomy can be performed as an office procedure. It must be emphasized that the operation does not affect the ability to achieve and sustain an erection, to achieve ejaculation, or to feel pleasure. There may be temporary minor swelling and pain in about half of those undergoing the procedure; these after-effects are successfully treated by applying an ice pack to the area to reduce the swelling, by temporarily using an athletic supporter, and by taking pain medication.

The effectiveness of the operation is evaluated by the physician's examination of ejaculates under the microscope for a period of several months afterwards. Two specimens, a month apart, both testing negative for sperm, is an accepted criterion for success. Some controversy exists among surgeons as to the precise techniques to be employed both for effective sterilization and to allow restoration of the male reproductive ducts, should this be desired at some later date.

Failure of vasectomy, as evidenced by viable sperm in ejaculates or an unwanted pregnancy at some time after the procedure, may result either from an inadequate surgical interruption of the vas or its later recanalization—an attempt by nature to repair the damage. Despite such considerations, one highly respected surgeon has reported no failures among more than 5,000 procedures he personally performed. Another prominent surgeon has indicated 97 failures, early and late, among an equally large number of patients. The latter results, however, are less disturbing in light of the fact that among the "technical failures" (presence of sperm on microscopic examination), no pregnancies resulted, and among the group as a whole, followed over a 20-year period, only four unwanted pregnancies occurred.

SEXUALLY TRANSMITTED DISEASES (STDS)

The table below lists the major sexually transmitted diseases (STDs) affecting American men. It also lists current estimates (male and female combined) of the known total incidence of each. Additionally, some 1.5 million Americans are believed to be infected with **HIV**, the human immunodeficiency virus, which is responsible for **AIDS** (acquired immune deficiency syndrome). AIDS is transmitted in three primary ways: sexually, by the use of contaminated hypodermic needles, and in blood

Major Sexually Transmitted Diseases in the United States*

Gonorrhea	1,400,000
Syphilis	100,000
Genital herpes	200,000 to 500,000
Chlamydia	4,000,000
Nonspecific urethritis	1,200,000
Hepatitis B	200,000
Human papilloma virus	500,000 to 750,000
Trichomoniasis	3,000,000

*Figures from the Centers for Disease Control, Atlanta

transfusions. (Current screening techniques and regulation of blood donors have reduced the risk of acquiring AIDS from blood transfusions to a minimum.)

Other venereal infections, such as **lymphogranuloma venereum, chancroid**, and **granuloma inguinale**, are not common enough to be considered major health problems. Hepatitis, although not ordinarily considered a sexually transmitted disease, can be acquired in this manner and is discussed later in that context.

Gonorrhea

For a man, the risk of acquiring gonorrhea from a single contact with an infected partner has been estimated at 17 percent. However, both men and women can harbor asymptomatic infections and be perfectly capable of transmitting the disease to a sex partner, with neither partner aware that one or the other of the two is infected. Can you contract gonorrhea from a contaminated toilet seat? In actuality, the gonococcus cannot live long upon exposure to the drying effect of air (although when smeared in pus on a toilet seat experimentally, it has survived for several hours). In purely practical terms, therefore, the acquisition of a gonococcal infection is always assumed to have been the result of intimate sexual contact.

Variations in the clinical picture of gonorrheal infection are now well recognized. Infections in the pharynx may occur after oral sex; involvement of the anus or rectum may occur among persons practicing anal intercourse. Any infected person may experience a disseminated infection with high fevers, pains, and occasionally prominent swelling of one or more joints, the last occurring in approximately one out of every 300 to 600 cases of gonorrhea.

Pelvic inflammatory disease, with fever and lower abdominal pain, is the female counterpart, and in both sexes repeated infections can result in scarring of the reproductive ducts, resulting in eventual sterility.

Symptoms. Typically the bacterial infection in men is heralded by symptoms of urethral inflammation, with pain and burning on urination. This is usually accompanied by a discharge of pus three to 10 days after intercourse with an infected partner. The epididymis may be involved in 10 to 30 percent of cases, and some patients may develop symptoms of epididymitis alone (swelling and pain in the back part of the scrotum).

Diagnosis. Diagnosis in men is usually simple; the offending microorganism is identifiable on stained smears of the discharge or specific culturing of the gonococcus in the laboratory. In the past it was recommended that all patients with gonorrhea undergo blood testing for concurrent asymptomatic syphilis, but, given the small number of hidden syphilis cases that this testing revealed, the value of this practice seemed questionable. At present it is probably most helpful to perform such testing among men and women with extensive numbers of sexual contacts.

Treatment. Penicillin is an initially easy and effective treatment for gonorrhea, and it still remains the drug of choice, except in allergic individuals. However, an increasing number of gonococcal strains resistant to penicillin are now being reported—between 1 and 3 percent of all cases, with the incidence tending to be higher in areas where the disease is most common. Fortunately, newer antibiotic regimens have been developed that are effective even in these cases. More selective and responsible sex, prompted by the fear of AIDS, has had a salutary effect in the control of gonorrheal spread. After a peak incidence in 1985 in the United States, new cases of gonorrhea have fallen 32 percent among heterosexual men and 48 percent among women.

Nongonococcal Urethritis

Over the last two decades it has become increasingly apparent that the majority of cases of acute urethritis (inflammation of the urethra) occurring in men were not due to the gonococcus, but rather were instances of nongonococcal urethritis. These now constitute the most rapidly growing STDs in men, rivaling even the growth of herpes. This trend has been worldwide, with a study in England and Wales demonstrating that by 1980 the incidence of nongonococcal urethritis was more than double that of gonococcal infections.

Some cases of nongonococcal urethritis have been found to be related to a microorganism called *Chlamydia trachomatis*. Others are still of uncertain cause.

Chlamydial urethritis. As might be suspected from its name, *C. trachomatis* is the organism responsible for trachoma, a major cause of blindness especially in the Middle East, North Africa, and northern India. Forms of this organism are also responsible for **lymphogranuloma venereum**, a relatively rare type of venereal disease in this country. In modern western societies its major importance lies in the fact that certain strains cause an STD with symptoms very similar to those of gonorrhea.

Recognition of chlamydial urethritis was initially delayed because of the small size of this bacterium. It is so small that at one time it was considered a virus. Recent improvements in laboratory diagnosis are now facilitating the diagnosis of chlamydia infection, which may be responsible for 40 to 50 percent of all cases of nongonococcal urethritis.

Fortunately, treatment of chlamydial infections is simple and effective; the antibiotics **tetracycline** and **erythromycin** are the drugs prescribed by most physicians in treating this infection.

Other types of nongonococcal urethritis. After gonorrhea and chlamydia, a considerable number of urethritis cases fall under other categories. Of these, as many as 30 percent may be due to another microorganism, *Ureaplasma urealyticum*, which is usually sensitive to tetracycline and similar drugs. In only about 1 to 2 percent are there other clearly identifiable causes—trichomonas, herpes, and fungal infections—leaving the majority of the nongonococcal, nonchlamydial urethritis cases unexplained.

It should be recognized that all cases of urethritis are not necessarily venereal in nature. **Reiter's syndrome**, a disease with urethritis, arthritis, and eye involvement, may follow sexual intercourse, but it has also been known to occur following episodes of gastroenteritis. Although various microorganisms have been shown to be involved in the genesis of Reiter's, the resulting symptoms are not due to acute bacterial infection but represent an autoimmune response. These cases are usually managed with anti-inflammatory medications. Although Reiter's is believed to be the most common type of inflammatory joint disease in young men, it probably represents no more than 2 to 3 percent of the total number of men complaining of urethritis.

Syphilis

No longer the scourge it was when it first broke out in epidemic proportions in sixteenth-century Europe, syphilis remains a formidable challenge because of its persistence throughout the world, its occasional transmission along with other more common venereal diseases, and the potentially lethal nature of its effects. Called "the great imitator," syphilis can ultimately affect any number of organ systems. Before Dr. Paul Ehrlich's "magic bullet" treatment (the arsenical Salvarsan), and later the introduction of penicillin, syphilis was the cause of major illness in large numbers of hospitalized patients.

Symptoms. The disease is caused by an organism called a **spirochete** because of its corkscrew appearance under the microscope. It occurs in a primary stage that quickly resolves itself, then may recur in a secondary and possibly a tertiary stage. The spirochete enters the body during intercourse. After a period of 10 to 30 days, ordinarily, a reddish spot forms on the shaft or tip of the penis. This swells into a **papule** (lump) that often breaks down into a painless ulcer, the syphilitic **chancre.** This primary form of the disease may be accompanied by swelling of lymph nodes in the groin. The patient may complain of oral or anal chancres, depending upon his sexual practices. Among women the primary chancre may often be relatively asymptomatic and hidden within the vagina. Untreated, the chancre will disappear after two to four weeks. This spontaneous resolution may represent the end of the disease or simply a step along the way to its secondary or tertiary forms.

Secondary syphilis usually begins six to eight weeks following exposure. It begins as a flulike illness with fever, generalized aches, and lymph-node enlargement. The characteristic feature of secondary syphilis is its rash, which, unlike most other generalized rashes, prominently involves the palms and soles. How long the rash lasts varies considerably. Again, this stage may represent the end of the story or just another intermediate step in the progression to a dreadful final stage of the disease. Syphilis can be transmitted from one partner to the other during the first or second stages. The third stage is noninfectious.

Tertiary or late syphilis may occur between three and 10 years following the initial infection. It may show up as a tumor (or **gumma**) in many parts of the body, but has a special predilection for the central nervous system—brain and spinal cord—and the cardiovascular system. It was the latter two types of involvement that accounted for so much morbidity and mortality in the medical wards of the past.

Diagnosis. Diagnosis of syphilis in the first stage can be made by obtaining swabs from the chancre and identifying the spirochete under the microscope. In the second stage, the spirochete may be obtained from the skin lesions, especially when the latter are "weeping." Essentially, though, all infected individuals' blood tests for the disease will now be positive, and this is the method of diagnosis usually employed. In screening for syphilis, the initial blood test that shows up positive may be in error (biologically false-positive) and further, more specific testing is indicated. Part of the clinical difficulty in diagnosing the infected patient involves the fact that either the first or second stage of the disease may not appear or may be missed clinically. It is estimated that of all those infected, about 30 percent of those untreated will ultimately go on to develop the final or tertiary stage of the disease.

Treatment. Penicillin is still effective when treating the primary and secondary stages of syphilis. Although the antibiotic is also administered if tertiary syphilis is diagnosed, the efficacy of therapy at this time is questionable. By this time, substantial damage to the involved organs has probably already occurred.

Genital Herpes

This disease, caused by the **herpes simplex** virus, has become one of the most distressing of STDs despite the fact that, except in newborns delivered of mothers with active lesions, the infection carries with it essentially no risk of death or permanent disability. Genital herpes infections constitute about 5 percent of all STDs reported by VD clinics, although this probably represents an underestimation of the numbers among males. Among college students, for example, genital herpes infections have been found to be 10 times more common than those of syphilis or gonorrhea. A recent survey, reported in 1989, indicated that with blood testing for antibodies to Type 2 herpes virus, 16.4 percent of Americans were positive, including many subclinical cases. The highest prevalence, 20.2 percent, was in the group 30 to 44 years of age.

Symptoms. Two types of herpes simplex have been identified and two patterns of disease involvement: **primary** and **recurrent.** Type 1 herpes is usually associated with oral infections of a nonvenereal type, though oral sex can infect a partner's genital area with Type 1 herpes. Someone afflicted with the initial Type 1 infection may experience fever and a general malaise, along with the development of painful ulcers in the mouth or lesions around the lips; these are known popularly as "cold sores" or "fever blisters." Although these heal within a week or so, the virus remains within the tissue, intact though dormant. It is reactivated by stressful physical conditions such as exposure to strong sunlight, wind, other infections, and perhaps mental distress. The skin lesions then reappear, but usually without other signs of illness.

Of major concern here are the Type 2 herpes infections, the type involved in most genital infections. Can genital herpes be acquired nonsexually—from spas, for instance? Although theoretically possible, such occurrences are rather unlikely. But the risk of acquiring the infection by intercourse with an infected individual actively shedding the virus is believed to be as high as 90 percent.

Following the primary genital herpes infection, there is an incubation period of from two to seven days. Tiny blisters, called **vesicular lesions,** then appear on the tip, shaft, or base of the penis. These blisters are usually painful and/or itchy and in about 40 percent of such cases may be accompanied by systemic signs of illness such as fever, sensitivity to light, and generalized aches and pains. In about half of the men affected, there may be a urethral discharge, and in the majority the initial bout will be accompanied by swelling of lymph nodes in the groin.

Diagnosis. The diagnosis can often be made within minutes in the doctor's office, both through the clinical appearance of the patient and by the physician's obtaining scrapings from the base of the lesions. These are placed on a slide, stained, and observed under the microscope. This inspection will identify the swollen cells characteristic of herpes, but will not differentiate between the two types. Since recurrent herpes is more common in Type 2 infections, blood testing to distinguish between the two is helpful for prognostic reasons. An internist, urologist, or dermatologist can make the diagnosis.

Treatment. After about two weeks, the primary infection, similar to Type 1 infections in the mouth, will subside spontaneously. If the drug **acyclovir** (Zovirax) is applied topically following the appearance of the lesions, the course may be shortened by three or four days; if it is given in capsule form by mouth, the time course of the primary infection may be cut in half.

Recurrent herpes. When genital herpes recurs, general and localized symptoms tend to be somewhat less severe than those accompanying a primary infection. The usual time course of the recurrence also tends to be shorter, about 10 days. The major hardship associated with recurrent genital herpes is psychological; the individual never knows when his life will be disrupted by new outbreaks of the disease. In those who have recurrences, the frequency may vary from as often as once a month to as infrequently as less than once every six months. However, the overall recurrence rate is about 60 percent, and recurrences tend to be more common in men than in women. The causes differ from person to person. In some patients, it is sunlight exposure that leads to new outbreaks of the sores; others react to fever or to minor irritation in the genital area; others claim emotional factors, which may or may not be the real cause. In many recurrences, no inciting factor can be identified.

The emotional stress that recurrent herpes can impose on a sexual relationship is severe, and various approaches to alleviating this stress have been attempted. Condoms offer some protection to your partner, but failures have been documented, especially when sheepskin rather than latex types have been employed. Moreover, there is always the problem of dislodgment of the condom during or immediately after the sex act. In general, it's best to refrain from intercourse during recurrent outbreaks, in order to avoid anxiety about possibly spreading the herpes virus to the uninfected partner.

Long-term use of acyclovir, with courses of therapy up to four years, have been shown to suppress recurrences of genital herpes in as many as 80 to 90 percent of cases. A six-month course of treatment is currently recommended. When recurrences do appear during this therapy, they seem to be comparatively milder and shorter. In some cases, where there has already been a prolonged course of acyclovir, no new recurrences appear when the drug is discontinued. Acyclovir, even when prescribed over long periods, seems to be well tolerated by most people. However, resistant herpes strains have now appeared, and other treatments are being investigated.

Pubic Lice

Lice that are limited to the pubic region are commonly called "crabs." They are almost always caused by sexual contact with an infected partner—who may or may not have symptoms of an infestation—although occasionally the source is infected bedding, clothing, or other items that contain the lice or their eggs.

Symptoms. The characteristic symptom is one of intense itching. The lice themselves are smaller than a pinhead. Though occasionally visible to the naked eye, they may better be seen with the aid of a magnifying glass. Easier to detect than the lice themselves are dark spots just under the skin, which may represent coagulated blood from their bites or their feces. The eggs (or nits) can sometimes be seen attached to the pubic hairs.

Treatment. Treatment is usually simple and effective. It involves shampooing with or applying an agent such as **lindane** (Kwell). Although neurological symptoms ranging from dizziness to convulsions have been described following the use of this drug on some people, these have almost always been related to accidental oral ingestion. Skin rashes due to allergy are also quite rare. In addition, clothes and bedding that have been in contact with the pubic area should be washed in hot water and dried on a hot dryer cycle to prevent reinfestation.

Hepatitis

Although not ordinarily thought of as an STD, hepatitis can be transmitted through sexual contact. Two forms of hepatitis have been generally recognized in the past: so-called **infectious**

hepatitis and **serum hepatitis.** The infective agent responsible for most cases of infectious hepatitis is a virus usually transmitted to humans by contaminated sewage, uncooked tainted foods, and other unsanitary conditions. This virus is known as **hepatitis A.** A second form of hepatitis, serum hepatitis, is so called because it is usually associated with the transfusion of contaminated blood products or as a result of the use of improperly sterilized hypodermic needles or surgical instruments. It is found in most cases to be associated with a different virus, **hepatitis B.**

Viral infections of the liver that cannot be shown to be the result of either hepatitis A or hepatitis B are now called **non-A/non-B** infections. It is now generally acknowledged that most of the non-A/non-B category probably represents infections with the recently isolated **hepatitis C** virus, although there are other, rarer types. Because of effective screening of donors who might harbor hepatitis A or B, the non-A/non-B strain has become the most common hepatitis related to blood transfusions.

Sexual transmission. In terms of sexual activity, it is the hepatitis B virus that is of paramount importance. There are several reasons for this. The course of hepatitis B infections is often more severe than hepatitis A infections, and about 2 percent of those hospitalized with acute hepatitis B will die. In contrast, recovery from hepatitis A infection is usually uneventful. Furthermore, whereas recovery from hepatitis A is complete, between 6 and 10 percent of those with hepatitis B become chronic carriers of the virus. In some of this group the infection will slowly progress as **chronic active hepatitis,** leading to long-term illness with complications of liver failure months or years later, often with fatal results. Finally, chronic hepatitis B infection leads to an increased susceptibility to liver cancer. In Asia, Africa, and other parts of the world where large numbers of people are infected, patients appear with this usually incurable form of cancer in the prime of life.

The recognition of the sexual mode of transmission for hepatitis B was one of the later findings during public-health efforts to limit the disease. In the process of screening blood donors as possible asymptomatic carriers of hepatitis B in New York City, it was found that many gay men with no previous knowledge of ever having hepatitis—no jaundice, swelling of the liver, dark urine, or other common symptoms of the disease—were testing positive for antibodies to hepatitis B.

When this group was looked at systematically in the mid-1970s, it turned out that the rate for positivity among gay men was 10 times that of heterosexual males. Trauma of the anus or rectum during anal intercourse, with even minor abrasions in the recipient, apparently allows virus in the semen of the partner to enter the bloodstream. When a vaccine to protect against infection with hepatitis B became available and needed a prospective trial, a group of uninfected gay men, followed over a period of months, proved ideal for this purpose. More than 1,000 entered the trial in New York, where half received the vaccine and half a placebo. It was demonstrated incontrovertibly that the vaccine offered highly effective protection for those who had received it. The vaccine itself is remarkably free from harmful side effects.

A final note on the sexual transmission of hepatitis: It is the group of viruses called non-A/non-B that are now achieving prominence. Currently about 10 percent of those with hepatitis contracted as a result of sexual contact are infected with this strain. Some of these may develop a form of hepatitis that is chronic, though usually not as severe as hepatitis B.

Symptoms. What is the course of hepatitis B? The incubation period (i.e., the time elapsing between the introduction of the virus and the appearance of symptoms) is rather long as well as variable, between 50 and 160 days. Flulike symptoms of fatigue, headache, and joint pain that persist for up to a week or two represent the onset; these are followed by the appearance of jaundice, darkening of the urine, and swelling of the liver with associated tenderness. In many patients, however, the disease may be mild and unaccompanied by any clinical jaundice, and thus go unrecognized and untreated.

Treatment. Currently it is recommended that hepatitis B vaccine be offered to sexually active gay men, intravenous drug abusers, and their spouses, and to certain health-care workers who run the risk of contact with infected blood through accidental needle sticks, cuts, and other hazards of their profession. For those who have already been exposed to contaminated blood or other body fluid of an infected person, vaccine (which stimulates the patient's body to produce antibodies after a time) should be preceded by **immune globulin** injections that contain antibodies immediately available to destroy the infecting virus.

AIDS

In the summer of 1981 the Centers for Disease Control in Atlanta noticed a pattern of hitherto unusual diseases appearing in young gay men. One was a type of pneumonia caused by a parasite, *Pneumocystis carinii,* an organism that had previously been known to exist primarily in cancer patients whose immune systems had been compromised as a result of chemotherapy. The other disease was a rare form of skin cancer, **Kaposi's sarcoma,** also very unusual in patients of this age group and general physical condition.

These patients were found to have markedly diminished numbers of particular white blood cells (**T helper lymphocytes**). Their affliction initially was called GRID (gay-related immune deficiency syndrome). Soon a demographic pattern developed among those afflicted with these and similar manifestations, and it became clear that not only gay men were affected.

We now know that the population base at risk for AIDS is much wider than was first believed. For example, non-drug-using female partners of male intravenous drug users can acquire the disease through sexual contact. When infected, they can pass it on to their newborn children. In fact, heterosexual contacts constitute the major transmission mode in parts of Africa where the disease has reached truly pandemic proportions. Rarely, health-care workers may be infected through handling of contaminated body fluids of patients with AIDS, the virus gaining entrance through needle sticks, finger cuts, or other open lesions on the body of the nurse, doctor, or medical technician.

The medical literature regarding the causes, effects, epidemiology, treatment, and basic research in this disease has literally exploded. The mass of new information emerging is so great that any publication more than a few weeks old may already be outdated.

Human immunodeficiency virus (HIV). The disease we call AIDS is the result of a virus called human immunodeficiency virus 1 (HIV-1), and is therefore frequently referred to in medical circles as **HIV disease.** Far less frequently the syndrome may be caused by a related virus, HIV-2, but at present this is of no broad practical significance.

The disease carries the descriptive term *immunodeficiency* because the virus appears to attack, among other cells, T lymphocytes, white blood cells prominently involved in helping the body resist infection. Patients ultimately appear with so-called opportunistic infections, those caused by organisms that other people, with normally functioning immune systems, have no difficulty resisting. The virus may also attack certain organs directly.

As already indicated, the virus gets into the bloodstream of its new victim. One early recognized route was through transfusions of infected blood (e.g., to hemophiliacs). Among intravenous drug users, shared contaminated needles are the vehicle of transmission. Among gay men, the virus enters the bloodstream through anal intercourse. Among heterosexuals the link is less clearly established (anal intercourse, vaginal sores) but transmission through such contact is undeniable. The risk to health-care personnel is real, but infection through this kind of contact is probably quite rare.

One insidious aspect of the disease is that it can be present without symptoms for months or, more likely, years. During this time, those infected can transmit the virus even though they feel and look perfectly well. It is only when an individual develops full-blown AIDS, perhaps five to seven years or more after being infected, that he becomes his own marker for the disease for others to recognize. As a consequence, it may be difficult to know if you have been in contact with an HIV-positive person.

How common is AIDS in the United States? A recent bulletin (1989) indicates that the number of AIDS cases reported since 1981 exceeds 100,000. Although absolute percentages vary from one locale to another, gay males and bisexuals as well as intravenous drug users are identified as the groups at highest risk. Recently, female partners of intravenous drug users, their newborns, and male and female prostitutes are receiving increased attention. With the screening of blood transfusions for viral antibodies and the rejection of high-risk groups as donors, infection by transfusion has been brought well under control.

What concerns each of us is our own risk of infection, given age, gender, and possible indulgence in "risky" behavior. Considering the recent advent of the disease, its long delay in manifesting itself, and no broad-based programs for routine detection, such figures are hard to come by. Increased sexual promiscuity, whether heterosexual—especially involving the frequent use of prostitutes—or homosexual, carries with it increased risk of acquiring an HIV infection. As testing for HIV among intravenous drug users becomes more widespread, we may find the rate of infection even higher among this group than among gay men. Among all AIDS cases in the United States, the number of cases among heterosexual, monogamous men who do not inject drugs continues to be exceedingly small.

Symptoms. Certain clinical categories have been defined within the spectrum of HIV infection. A relatively mild, flulike illness with some swelling of the lymph nodes may occur within weeks of an infection, but this is often so minor it is overlooked. There is a long period, usually years, during which the virus is present and the patient is without symptoms, yet can infect other people. It is believed that in the majority of these cases, full-blown AIDS will eventually develop. The best current estimate is that this will happen in up to 70 percent of all those infected within 10 years of the initial infection.

Between the asymptomatic carrier state and the symptomatic state, two intermediate stages have been identified. One is **chronic lymphadenitis syndrome,** defined as the finding of swollen lymph nodes in at least two areas *other* than the groin (or inguinal) region for a period of three months or more. Those in the groin area are discounted because so many healthy people have palpable nodes there.

The other intermediate syndrome is **AIDS-related complex (ARC).** Patients with ARC will have many of the general symptoms of AIDS patients—weight loss, fatigue, fevers, swollen lymph nodes—but without the presence of any of the opportunistic infections or cancers characteristic of AIDS.

In fully developed AIDS, infections start to appear, the lung infection **Pneumocystis carinii pneumonia (PCP)** being the most common. Other infections, some until recently only of textbook interest because of their previous rarity, show up with some regularity in AIDS patients. These include **cryptococcal infection** (usually meningitis), **toxoplasmosis** in the brain, and tuberculosis in its ordinary form and in a rare form called **Mycobacterium avium intracellulare** that seems to be resistant to the drugs usually effective in ordinary TB. The fungal infection **candidiasis** often appears as white patches in the mouth ("oral thrush") and involves the esophagus, making swallowing difficult. Another serious viral infection, **cytomegalous virus** (CMV), may be life-threatening in about 8 percent of AIDS patients, affecting predominantly the gastrointestinal tract, lungs, and eyes. In addition to these unusual infections, AIDS patients are also more susceptible to the many ordinary microorganisms that cause disease among the general population.

Certain types of unusual cancers are also relatively frequent among AIDS patients. Kaposi's sarcoma may appear in the skin or internally and, for reasons not well understood, is far more common among gay male AIDS patients than among intravenous drug users. A fairly difficult-to-treat lymph node malignancy, **non-Hodgkins lymphoma,** also has a high incidence among AIDS patients.

The virus may attack certain tissues directly. The brain and the heart are especially susceptible areas.

Diagnosis. How can AIDS be diagnosed? When the full-blown syndrome of AIDS, with its generalized symptoms, infections, and cancers, occurs in patients within high-risk groups, the picture is so typical that blood testing is often merely a formality. The real challenge involves detection of the many patients who are carrying the virus and have yet to develop the clinical disease we call AIDS.

As is typical with all viral infections, there is a period during which the virus reproduces itself and specific antibodies are produced in the body in response to it. Current laboratory testing can spot the antibodies produced by the infection rather than the virus itself. The **ELISA test** (enzyme-linked immunoabsorbent assay) and the **Western Blot test** are commonly used and are usually performed in that order for screening purposes. Both are quite sensitive and highly reliable in laboratories devoted to this kind of work. But false-positive findings may occur when the tests are not performed with care, or in less experienced laboratories.

Because of the devastating medical and social consequences of a positive test for HIV, any positive ELISA should be followed by a repeat of the test. Two positive ELISAs should then be confirmed by the Western Blot test.

Although this may seem a rather clear-cut approach to the diagnosis of HIV infection, it is far from a simple matter. The problem lies in the time that elapses between infection and the appearance within the bloodstream of antibodies that can be detected by either of the above tests. This latency period is extremely variable. In some patients, antibodies will appear within a matter of weeks; in others, as recently shown in a prospective study of high-risk sexually active gay men, it may take as long as two to four years for HIV to result in detectable antibody levels.

Why not test the blood for the virus directly, instead of waiting for antibodies to appear? Although not generally available as of this writing, one such test for early detection has been devised and may soon become routine in HIV testing. It uses **polymerase,** an enzyme that provokes rapid duplication of minute amounts of viral DNA within a test tube, thus eliminating the need to wait for antibodies to the virus to appear in the blood. For the present, however, the bottom line is that your sexual partner may be infected with the virus and capable of transmitting it, and neither you nor your partner may be aware of it.

Treatment. Because there is no specific cure for AIDS, primary efforts for AIDS patients currently are directed toward the control and elimination of opportunistic infections. The most common of these infections and the leading cause of death among AIDS patients is PCP. The sulfa drug **Bactrim** is effective in the treatment of this acute infection. **Pentamidine** has more recently been shown to be effective for acute infections, and is the drug of choice in prophylaxis and prevention of recurrent infections. But over time the effectiveness of these drugs seems to wear off, and the patient succumbs to the illness. Other identifiable infective microorganisms may be susceptible to various other antibiotic regimens. Chemotherapy and radiation are used to treat Kaposi's sarcoma and non-Hodgkins lymphoma.

When the heart is involved, appropriate drugs may be used to assist its function. When the destructive effects of the virus focus on the brain, little more than supportive care can be provided.

At present there is no curative drug to eliminate the virus, and no vaccine to prevent its infecting new patients. AZT (Zidovudine, Retrovir) has been shown to decrease both mortality and the numbers of recurrent opportunistic infections in those already infected. It does not provide a cure and can have serious side effects, among them a reduction of red cells (causing anemia) and certain white blood cells other than T lymphocytes. Fortunately, recent studies show that lower doses of AZT are equally effective and may reduce the risk of this side effect.

At present, intense evaluation of other therapeutic agents is being undertaken. Steroids, usually considered harmful in the presence of infection, have been shown to assist the effectiveness of treatment in PCP. Following encouraging studies in laboratory animals, a vaccine trial for HIV infection is now under way. Still, death continues to occur relatively swiftly and universally following a case of full-blown AIDS. A study of nearly 6,000 AIDS cases in New York City showed the overall probability of survival to be 49 percent at one year and 15 percent at five years after the onset of the disease.

Prevention. Because of the current unsatisfactory status of medical treatment for AIDS, prevention of the infection is the primary issue. "Safe sex" has become the byword in advice by physicians to their patients, and includes

- avoidance of sexual contact with those suspected of having AIDS or harboring the human immunodeficiency virus
- avoidance of anal intercourse
- limitation of the number of sexual contacts, with emphasis on the advantages of monogamous relationships
- avoidance of sexual contact with intravenous drug users

The use of condoms has been strongly advised for sexual intercourse, although their use does not confer absolute protection; the same limitations and drawbacks apply to AIDS prevention as apply to prevention of other sexually transmitted diseases.

Psychological, social, and economic effects. The rapid growth and impact of AIDS on our society is astounding. At first considered by many only an aberrant illness within narrow sectors of our society, AIDS stimulated more curiosity than concern. With its recognition as an incurable disease capable of infecting millions of people, AIDS has become a national and international problem involving all kinds of health-care personnel, governmental agencies, and private and public research centers. The many aspects of this problem, as they confront the individual and society as a whole, are inextricably entwined.

For the person with AIDS, there is the frightening awareness of an incurable illness and imminent death, almost always in the prime of life. The stigma of AIDS has not been removed by the fact that it now strikes a wider range of people. Jobs are lost, housing is denied, friends fade away, and even family may abandon the AIDS victim on his or her way to the inevitable end.

As heavy as this emotional burden is, it is not the only one. Hospitalizations are prolonged and involved, and financial resources are quickly depleted. The financial burden is soon shifted to the hospital caring for such patients. Even with governmental reimbursement programs in place, hospitalization of each AIDS victim can result in many thousands of dollars in unpaid bills, and many private hospitals, often on the brink of financial insolvency, now refuse to admit these patients.

As a result, many of the patients believe they are being ignored by their communities. Gay activists especially have campaigned, urging the development of new drugs and governmental programs. There has seemed to be, at times, an inordinate delay in testing and approving new drugs that hold out some promise in the treatment of AIDS. The truth is that it is precisely when no cure is available for a rapidly fatal disease that many quack remedies are introduced by the misguided or unscrupulous, and accepted by the desperate and gullible. Evaluation of new drugs is a time-consuming and tedious business. Whether or not the Food and Drug Administration (FDA) may have dragged its feet in the past, recent activity at the federal level suggests that the agency is now moving as quickly as possible to test new AIDS drugs.

It must be understood that very few viruses can be killed by medications once the virus has entered the body. The major advances in the control of previous viral diseases have been in immunology, through the development of effective vaccines. Here we are dealing with an extremely elusive retrovirus that enters the nucleus of the victim's cells and incorporates itself as part of the cells' own DNA until the time it emerges and makes it presence known as the disease we recognize as AIDS. Not only can HIV disguise itself, but it has also shown a great ability to mutate, thus presenting a shifting target for any vaccine devised against it.

Ethical issues. Even getting a firm epidemiological grip on AIDS is a daunting prospect. Who should be tested? How often? Why? Given the devastating social consequences of being labeled HIV-positive, and the lack of a cure, legitimate questions are raised about the value of such testing, despite all the safeguards for confidentiality and anonymity that are in place.

Yet some AIDS experts are now making convincing arguments for testing those who suspect that they may be harboring the organism. Evidence is accumulating that if treatment is provided *before* the onset of clinical AIDS, it might forestall the symptoms and even prolong life. Furthermore, personal awareness of infection can lead to protective measures not only for patients themselves, but for their loved ones and the community as a whole.

Hysteria about AIDS is not limited to the lay public. Even today, many health-care workers refuse to care for AIDS patients, and precautions taken by nurses and doctors alike are often excessive in the absence of potential harmful contact.

As for the future, despite improved efforts to control AIDS through public and personal health measures, the disease, with all its frightening aspects, will be with us long into the foreseeable future, and probably without an effective cure. Although this is disheartening, some comfort may be gleaned from the fact that so much has been learned so quickly. Diseases such as syphilis and paralytic polio afflicted many for hundreds of years without the cause being known, much less a cure discovered. Within 10 years, medical scientists have learned an impressive amount about HIV. We must remain hopeful that before too long a preventive—perhaps even a cure—will emerge.

OTHER SEXUALLY TRANSMITTED DISEASES

Besides the major STDs, there are a number of other infections that can affect the sexually active male. Some are less serious than others, and most can be prevented by the use of a condom during intercourse.

Trichomoniasis. A common protozoal infection primarily affecting women, this one-celled parasite often causes itching and a vaginal discharge. In men it is occasionally a cause of urethritis, but it may be present in either sex without causing symptoms. Once diagnosed, the disease is easily treated with the drug **metronidazole** (Flagyl), but if reinfection occurs it may be necessary for both partners to undergo a course of therapy. Although usually transmitted during sex, the organisms can survive in a moist environment and therefore may be passed on through wet towels, damp bathing suits, or locker room benches.

Lymphogranuloma venereum. This is another facet of *Chlamydia trachomatis* infection in humans (see page 137). Strains responsible for this type of infection first cause a stage of lymph gland swelling, and later on a generalized illness that may include fever, chills, muscle aches, and joint involvement. Although common in many Third World countries, it is relatively rare in the United States.

Chancroid. Another relatively rare STD in this country, this bacterial infection causes painful ulcerations on the genitalia.

Genital warts. These are caused by the human papilloma virus (HPV). Although unsightly, they usually cause no symptoms and can be removed with a laser in the dermatologist's office. The major significance of this virus is that HPV has been incriminated as a causative element in several cancers of the genital tract and anus, primarily cervical cancer in women.

If You Think You Have an STD

Since the risk of acquiring STDs increases with every new partner, there is a growing trend among heterosexuals and gays alike to make their sexual relationships monogamous. But the reality remains that no matter how discerning you wish to be, you cannot be sure that a potential partner is free of disease.

He or she may be totally without symptoms and yet perfectly capable of transmitting a disease to you.

What to look for. For the sexually active male, *some* risk of venereal infection always exists. When infection occurs or is suspected, medical assistance should be sought as soon as possible. If you observe any of the following symptoms, see a doctor immediately.

A **whitish discharge** from the penis, especially when accompanied by pain or burning, suggests gonorrhea. The diagnosis can usually be made at the doctor's office. In the absence of gonorrhea, chlamydial infection is likely. Ureaplasma infection, trichomonas, and Reiter's syndrome are much less likely to be the cause. In a substantial number of cases of urethritis, no specific cause may be identified.

A **sore** or **ulceration** on the penis should raise considerations of syphilis, or chancroid if the lesion is solitary. Most commonly, a cluster of herpetic vesicular lesions or blisters is a good reason to seek medical help. Frequently overlooked by the anxious patient is the possibility that a penile lesion may not be venereal at all. An ulcer on the tip of the penis can result from frictional irritation; allergic reactions of the skin may involve the penis and scrotum; psoriasis and many other skin disorders may involve the genital area.

Sudden **swelling of lymph nodes** in the groin can be part of a generalized viral infection totally unrelated to sexual exposure to disease. Many people, especially those accustomed to walking in their bare feet outdoors, have chronically enlarged lymph nodes in the groin, probably related to numerous previous subclinical infections. These are no cause for concern. However, an acute enlargement of these nodes accompanied by a penile lesion suggests herpes or possible syphilis, and is a cause for concern.

A **rash** in the area of the genitals may be nonvenereal or venereal in nature. Contact dermatitis related to some allergen in newly acquired underwear or swimsuits can be the actual cause. Reaction to heat and moisture in this area can be manifested in a rash. Generalized rashes from any cause can include the genitals. Fungal infections can also appear in this area.

Sudden **itching** in the pubic area and neighboring parts after sexual exposure always suggests the possibility of pubic lice, or "crabs." Examination for evidence of this infestation, described previously, should settle the question.

Do not lose sight of the fact that even when STDs do occur in one or another of these guises, for the most part they can be successfully treated and, with proper precautions, are unlikely to cause permanent harm. The STDs that are real threats to survival—AIDS and, occasionally, hepatitis—do not present symptoms of typical venereal diseases.

A corollary to the early diagnosis and treatment of STDs in the individual is that all recent sexual contacts should be identified, informed, and encouraged to undergo necessary testing and treatment themselves. This may cause considerable stress between sexual partners, but only in this way can the chain of disease transmission be broken.

6

Mental and Emotional Health

Much has been written lately in the media and elsewhere about the impact of stress upon our mental and emotional stability. It's true that deaths of family members and friends, personal illness, marital problems, difficulties on the job, financial insecurity, and problems with one's children all pose major threats to our sense of well-being that we must all confront at one time or another in the course of our lives.

Most of us find ways to cope with such obstacles to happiness and fulfillment. When our own efforts fail, we may seek assistance from those trained in the evaluation and treatment of mental disorders and social maladjustments. In addition to problems of adjustment to life's pressures, there are, of course, serious mental illnesses that cause severe disability and require hospitalization and psychiatric treatment.

The terms *neurosis* and *psychosis* have been used historically to distinguish between two general classifications of mental disorder. Essentially, those afflicted with neurotic disorders maintain their sense of reality throughout the course of their disease. Psychotics, on the other hand, may experience delusions, visual or auditory hallucinations, and extremes of confusion and memory loss, not as troubling symptoms of their illness, but as reality. The neurotic patient frequently continues to function in society—going on with his or her daily work and household tasks despite any distress caused by mental or emotional symptoms. The psychotic patient, on the other hand, is characterized by social withdrawal and failure in his daily personal functioning.

MIDLIFE CRISIS IN MEN

With our gradually increasing life span, more men than ever before are now reaching what is considered midlife, the ages 50 to 65. With our improved ability to address our physical ills, more and more attention has come to be focused on the emotional life of men in these middle years. The various inner and external factors coming into play during this period have created what some have termed "male midlife crisis" and others have called "male menopause."

Unlike female menopause, no dramatic hormonal change takes place, so the term *menopause* is not physiologically appropriate for men. However, the stresses and strains of that time in life are no less meaningful for men.

Unfortunately, some men attempt to relieve those stresses through divorce, alcohol, or even attempts at suicide. Better to begin to enjoy the world in "more diffusely sensual ways," as the psychologist David Gutmann has put it. He defines this period of midlife reassessment as yet another phase of normal development in which certain adjustments need to be made.

This clear-sighted look at our past history and future options may be difficult for some men to achieve, but the human male is a more flexible animal than we sometimes think. Indeed, if he neglects this important passage of life, damaging emotional consequences can follow, such as acute anxiety attacks, depression, and other debilitating mental and emotional disorders.

ANXIETY DISORDERS

Anxiety and fear are normal reactions of the human experience. As such, we look upon these emotions as protective mechanisms—perceived warnings of danger that allow for effective solutions to deal with threats to our welfare. In psychiatric terms, however, fear is a normal response to a recognizable danger, while anxiety is a conscious reaction to an unconscious stimulus. In other words, anxiety is an abnormal reaction to a "danger" that is usually not perceived as such by others. Such anxiety is often "free-floating" in the sense that the sufferer himself may not be able to pinpoint just what it is he is afraid of.

Anxiety attacks. The manifestations of an anxiety attack are often expressed in physical terms—that is, in changes in certain bodily functions that are readily apparent to the patient and his physician. The primary focus can involve the cardiovascular system, with rapid heart rates producing a sense of palpitations or pressure in the chest. In other patients, gastrointestinal symptoms may be prominent, with diarrhea a common complaint. Blanching of the skin, sweating, or trembling may frequently accompany anxiety attacks.

Anxiety occasionally appears as hyperventilation. The individual overbreathes (usually unconsciously), blowing off excessive amounts of carbon dioxide. The resulting alkalosis (decreased acidity of the blood) may cause faintness, numbness, and tingling of the extremities and around the mouth. Or an oppressive tightness in the chest may provoke fear of a heart attack. Emergency-room physicians frequently encourage such anxiety-ridden patients to breathe and rebreathe into a paper bag in order to raise blood levels of carbon dioxide and thus alleviate these symptoms. Patients can learn to do this on their own when such symptoms recur, although, if anxiety attacks are persistent and/or severe, psychiatric counseling is advised.

Panic attacks. These represent another form of neurotic anxiety behavior. Here the onset is very sudden and severe, but usually short-lived. Attacks often occur about two or three times weekly. Panic disorders are common; it has been estimated that panic-attack victims make up 15 percent of those people initially consulting cardiologists, 25 percent of those visiting general practitioners, and between 5 and 25 percent of patients seeing psychiatrists. Although panic attacks can develop at any age, the average onset is at about age 25, with an equal distribution between men and women.

Phobias. These are a form of neurosis involving excessive and unreasonable fear of certain objects or situations. An abnormal fear of flying in a plane is one form, as is an excessive, paralyzing fear of heights. Acute fear of certain domestic animals (horses, dogs, cats), is another.

A specific type of phobia (also classified as a panic disorder) is **agoraphobia**—the fear of venturing out into open or public places. Symptoms of this phobia can progress to a point where the sufferer becomes an unwilling prisoner in his own home as a result of his fears. Certain drugs, combined with supportive psychotherapy, have been effective in restoring many such individuals to normal function.

In our culture, men are much more reluctant than women to complain about such disturbances as excessive anxiety, panic attacks, and phobias. Since effective treatment is available, men should be encouraged to seek psychiatric help rather than stoically attempt to brave it out on their own. Although standard psychotherapy may not be too helpful in treating phobias, many have found relief in behavioral therapy, which involves "thought stoppage" and other phobia-relieving techniques. Drug therapy has also helped some sufferers.

MOOD DISORDERS: DEPRESSION AND MANIA

Mood disorders constitute one of the most common types of disturbance seen in psychiatric practice. **Depression,** the most common, is at the low end of the spectrum, with characteristics similar to those suggested by the ordinary interpretation of the word. **Mania,** its opposite, refers to feelings of false elation, a sense of grandiosity and expansiveness. According to the American Psychiatric Association, when only depression *or* mania is exhibited by the patient, the disorder is called *unipolar;* where there are excessive swings of mood from one extreme to the other, it is called *bipolar*.

Mood refers to the inner feeling of the patient; *affect* is the external expression of the mood as it is observed by others. Thus the term *affective disorders* is still used to describe depression, mania, or a combination of the two.

Depression

It is estimated that 10 percent of men will, at some time in their lives, undergo at least one episode of severe depression. In about 50 percent of all patients seen (both men and women), the onset is usually between the ages of 20 and 50. The cause of the disorder is unknown, although there appears to be some genetic predisposition; depression is frequently found in the patient's family history. (Currently, two types of depressive disorder have been identified as related to specific chromosomes.) External factors such as anxiety and stress also play a role and can precipitate depressive episodes even in those who do not have familial propensities.

In general, the symptoms of depression include

- a predominant mood of sadness or withdrawal observed by the patient as well as by those around him
- a markedly diminished interest in pleasure; apathy
- a loss of appetite with resulting weight loss
- sleeplessness (insomnia) or its opposite, excessive sleeping
- agitation or sluggishness in physical reponses
- chronic fatigue
- feelings of worthlessness or guilt
- diminished ability to think clearly or decisively
- recurrent thoughts of death or suicide

Various combinations of these symptoms can lead to a diagnosis of depression, when there is no physical disease to account for them and no evidence of psychosis.

Although depressive illness is often cyclic, or tending to recur periodically, many effective therapies are available to treat acute episodes. Several drugs have been shown to be useful. The newest and currently the most popular of these is **fluoxetine** (Prozac). Although it has fewer side effects than the older antidepressants, it is not totally free of them: about 25 percent of users experience anxiety symptoms and, rarely, the drug may induce suicidal states. Antidepressants, however, are not addicting and may often be discontinued after six months of therapy. Psychotherapy is typically integrated with the drug regimen in the case of major depression.

A decision must be made in all cases of acute depression whether or not to admit the patient to the hospital. In view of the risk of suicide—approximately two-thirds of depressed patients contemplate suicide, and 10 to 15 percent successfully complete it—hospitalization can help.

Sadly, despite the devastating effects of depression and the availability of effective treatment, it is believed that only 20 to 25 percent of those affected ever seek treatment.

Mania and Manic Depression

Mania is characterized by feelings of extreme euphoria and grandiosity. During manic episodes those affected are talkative, show a decreased need for sleep, lack their normal inhibitions, are easily distracted, "race" through ideas, and are excessively physically active. Extreme irritability may also be part of the picture, and as many as three-quarters of such patients are often abusive or assaultive. Although not ordinarily considered a psychotic disorder, mania may be accompanied by delusions or hallucinations.

Manic episodes may occur without alternating periods of depression, but, more often, are part of a bipolar disorder formerly called **manic depression**. The overall lifetime risk of bipolar disease in men and women is almost equal at about one percent of the population.

Lithium remains a first-line drug for mania and depression in manic-depressive patients. Neurological, cardiac, and other side effects of this drug have been documented, gradually dampening the initial enthusiasm it generated when it was originally introduced more than 30 years ago. However, used in lower doses and, at times, in combination with other drugs, lithium has proved safe and especially effective in the treatment of severe and recurrent manic episodes.

In severe cases, when other medical treatment has failed, **electroconvulsive therapy** may be indicated. Although such therapy is one of the most effective treatments for severe depression, it has become controversial, involving as it does the use of electric shocks and the induction of seizures, both of which are frightening to the public and to the patient. But side effects are minimal today. Cardiovascular symptoms (extra beats and blood-pressure changes) are frequent but rarely serious. Bone fractures related to convulsions have been eliminated by use of muscle-relaxing agents. The most frequently reported long-term effect has been memory loss, which can be especially difficult to judge in patients whose underlying psychiatric dysfunction may include this symptom already. Recent careful studies have not substantiated long-term memory loss in patients, although temporary memory loss is common.

There is a growing feeling among psychiatrists that public revulsion has caused electroconvulsive therapy to be underutilized in recent years. They point to its rapid results in many drug-resistant patients.

Personality Disorders

Personality disorders, among the most common of psychiatric problems, are also among the most difficult to treat. Although frequently described in psychotic terms (paranoid, schizoid), such individuals have none of the defining characteristics of psychotics. Actually, they superficially resemble neurotics. However, patients with personality disorders, unlike neurotics, think of themselves as perfectly normal and rarely seek help for their problems. As a result, their patterns of behavior, well established by adolescence, usually persist throughout adulthood. There is evidence to indicate some genetic basis for such behavior patterns. In identical twins, for example, the possibility of a personality disorder existing in both twins is several times greater than in fraternal twins.

The different types of personality disorders are readily recognizable. All of us have encountered people suffering from one or another of them among our personal, social, or professional contacts.

- The **paranoid personality** is characterized by his long-standing suspicion and mistrust of others.

- The **schizoid personality** is isolated and lonely, but uncomfortable with human contact.
- **Histrionic** types are excitable, emotional, and flamboyant, but often superficial in their relationships.
- **Antisocial** subjects are unable to conform to the norms of society and are often found among the criminal class.
- **Narcissistic** personalities tend to focus on their own physical and personal attributes and problems to the exclusion of others.
- **Avoidant** personalities are unable to interact with others for fear of rejection, and are commonly labeled as having "inferiority complexes."
- The **dependent** personality is a submissive individual who often burdens others with his personal indecision and is in constant need of approval and reassurance from others.
- The **compulsive** person is characterized by his inflexibility and perfectionism as well as his indecisiveness.
- The **passive-aggressive** man is driven by an underlying aggression masked by subtle obstructionism, inefficiency, and resistance to change.
- The **sadistic** personality delights in hurting others.
- The **masochistic** individual enjoys being hurt or abused.

OTHER MENTAL DISORDERS

All of us know someone who is excessively fearful of overlooking some detail, who continually rechecks or repeats actions beyond any rational justification. An idea or an impulse continually intrudes itself upon the consciousness of this person, forcing him to take countermeasures against it and resulting in a disruption of his normal living patterns. He is often aware of the absurd nature of his acts (incessant hand washing, multiple trips back home to check the gas stove or electric lights). This condition is known as **obsessive-compulsive** disorder. Despite their distress, many such people will go on for years without seeking medical help. The onset of their symptoms occurs under the age of 35 in more than 80 percent of such patients, and the course is extremely variable.

For those seeking treatment, drugs provide some relief as long as they continue to be taken on a regular basis. Although usual forms of psychotherapy have not been too successful in treating obsessive-compulsive disorder, behavior modification techniques (see page 184) have shown some benefit.

Hypochrondriasis is a type of neurotic behavior characterized by excessive concern about disease and an intense preoccupation with one's health. Interestingly, it seems to be more common in men than in women, peaking between the fourth and fifth decades of life and representing between 5 and 15 percent of patients coming to medical doctors with physical complaints or concerns. Unfortunately, the long-term outlook, even with treatment, is not promising. Some two-thirds of these patients run a fluctuating course even when psychiatric assistance is accepted as part of the therapy.

The hypochondriac must not be looked upon as a malingerer, one who feigns disease to avoid work or other responsibilities. Nor should he be confused with the rare but deeply disturbed patient with the so-called **Baron Munchausen syndrome,** named after the eighteenth-century German nobleman and teller of tall tales. Although the psychodynamics of Baron Munchausen syndrome are poorly understood, people with this disorder will often go to extraordinary lengths to develop ways to feign certain diseases. Often they obtain hospital admission and even undergo treatment (sometimes including surgery!) before being discovered; they then appear later at another hospital where the same scenario is repeated.

A more commonly observed phenomenon is the secondary gain of physical illness observed among individual patients. Often easily recognized by the patient's family members as well as by the attending physician, secondary gain represents the gratification that the ill obtain from all the special attention lavished upon them during the course of their incapacitation. As a result, they unconsciously seek to prolong their illness to ensure a continuation of the special emotional rewards it has brought them.

PSYCHOSES

Disordered thinking, withdrawal, and a loss of a sense of reality characterize **psychoses.** Psychoses may often occur as a result of brain degeneration in the elderly, or as one result of the excessive use of drugs and alcohol.

About one percent of the population develops a type of psychosis called *schizophrenia.* Because of the onset of the disease early in life and the severity and difficulty of managing it, schizophrenics once accounted for a major proportion of those confined to large mental institutions. Though today attempts are made to release less severe cases for outpatient management, the disease still constitutes a baffling and often heartbreaking segment of mental illness in our society.

As with all psychoses, schizophrenia entails a loss of reality perception and an inability to function normally in society. Certain specific categories of the illness have been recognized for many years. These include the **disorganized** type (hebephrenic), characterized by infantile, primitive behavior and inappropriate emotional responses; the **catatonic** type, with marked symptoms of immobility; the **paranoid** type, with delusions of persecution. Finally there are those sufferers who do not fit neatly into these descriptions and so are collectively described as **undifferentiated.**

Although in the past schizophrenia has typically been resistant to drug therapy, new pharmacological agents have recently become available that appear promising. One of these is **remoxipride** and the other **clozapine** (Clozaril). Initial favorable results are being followed up with additional trials. However, a severe drop in white blood cell counts has been observed in 1 to 2 percent of those using the latter drug. This is a potentially life-threatening condition that requires constant monitoring of those under treatment with clozapine.

SUICIDE

Few among us have not been touched on at least one occasion by the suicide of someone close to us, or have had thoughts of suicide ourselves at one time or another. Or we may have been confronted by a distraught friend, relative, or acquaintance expressing thoughts of death.

Suicide is not a mental disease, but rather the tragic and final result of an inadequate diagnosis and treatment of a mental illness. Sometimes suicide is committed "rationally"—the terminal patient who no longer wishes to continue his suffering and disability comes to mind—but for the most part it is the end result of severe psychiatric illness. Predominantly this involves patients with affective disorders (manic depression), alcoholism and drug use, and schizophrenia.

Susan J. Blumenthal, M.D., of the National Institute of Mental Health, has studied this problem in depth and has attempted to define risk factors. Her work provides doctors with valuable help in assessing suicidal patients and establishing guidelines for timely and effective treatment. She states that as many as 50 percent of those who commit suicide have seen a doctor in the month prior to death, and that in the overwhelming majority of such encounters it was a nonpsychiatrist who was approached.

Dr. Blumenthal has identified five overlapping domains that help target the suicide-prone person: psychiatric diagnosis, personality traits or disorders, psychosocial and environmental factors (including medical illness), family history and genetics, and biological factors.

More than 90 percent of people committing suicide have some form of psychiatric illness, most often manic depression and alcoholism. Among the former, about 15 percent will end their lives in this way. (The scope of the problem becomes even more impressive when it is recognized that more than 10 million Americans suffer from depressive disorders.) Alcohol dependency is implicated in between 25 to 50 percent of suicides. Among alcoholics it is estimated that suicide will be the cause of death in 5 to 27 percent. Those who are drug-dependent have a 20 times higher risk of suicide than does the general population, and 15 percent of schizophrenics will end their lives in this way.

Basic personality problems are a second contributing factor. Suicidal victims are often antisocial in their behavior. Rigidity, accompanied by a strong element of hopelessness, is their response to the stresses of life.

Psychosocial and adverse environmental factors can also pre-cipitate suicide. Divorce, the threat of criminal prosecution, cha-otic family conditions, loss of a job, or other impending humiliation may drive the suicidally prone over the precipice. Among the elderly, the age group that constitutes the largest proportion of deaths by suicide, death of a mate or a severe debilitating illness may be the inciting factor.

Family history is an important element. The death of the novelist Ernest Hemingway by a self-inflicted gunshot wound, so similar to that of his father, is only one striking example of a pattern common in suicide victims. It has been shown that among psychiatric inpatients, 50 percent of those with a family history of suicide had attempted it themselves. Among the gen-eral population, 6 percent of successful suicides had a parent whose life had ended in the same way—88 times higher than that predicted among the general populace.

The danger here is that the death of a parent by suicide may set in motion a "self-fulfilling prophecy" to the offspring. Hem-ingway, for example, had long been morbidly fascinated by the suicide of his father, a successful physician, and this obsession may have driven him to end his life in the same way. Genetic factors may increase the statistical likelihood of suicide, but alteration of one's life-style, along with proper medical and psy-chiatric treatment, can very much even out the odds. For in-stance, biochemical investigations have revealed that a certain neurotransmitter, **serotonin,** is deficient in the brains of suicide victims, leading to the possibility that pharmaceutical ap-proaches to the problem may one day become practical and effective.

Physicians are attempting to become more adept at recogniz-ing the suicidally prone patient. For the individual at risk, and for those closely related to him, there are also many interven-tionist personal strategies such as risk clinics and telephone hot lines that are making some headway against this major problem.

SLEEP DISORDERS

Insomnia, the inability to fall asleep and obtain adequate rest, is one of the most common of human complaints. About one-third of Americans admit that acute insomnia has been a problem at some time during their lives. Although a frequent component of mental disorders, for the most part insomnia represents a minor disruption of our normal biological rhythms. This is most apparent in the phenomenon of jet lag among those who fly from one time zone to another, and among people like nurses and policemen who must frequently change their working shifts.

Although one often reads that we spend one-third of our lives in the sleeping state, the continuous eight-hour nightly rest is hardly a precise model. Enormous variability exists throughout the normal spectrum of sleep. At one end, a brilliant American scientist was known to begin his typical 14- or 15-hour day in the laboratory during the small hours of the morning. Many considered this an expression of his professional competitiveness, but he claimed that he never needed more than four hours of sleep a night. Like most biological phenomena, the normal sleeping curve is bell-shaped. At the ends are the few people who need either very little or very much sleep, with the greatest number collected at the seven-to-nine-hour-per-night portion of the curve.

Patterns of sleep may also vary. Some of the world's great achievers turn out to have been "nappers." Napoleon, Churchill, and Edison all compensated for a short night's sleep with a nap here and there during the day or evening.

Treating Insomnia

For those troubled by sleeplessness, it is important to recognize that no one ever died from lack of sleep. Although sleep deprivation in certain individuals has caused hallucinations, the final consequence is not psychosis but a collapse into a deep sleep.

After the first hour or two of sleep, a phase characterized by **rapid eye movement** (REM) intervenes. This lasts for about 90 minutes and recurs at regular intervals during the night. It is during REM sleep that dreams occur—whether or not we remember them—and it is this type of slumber that some experts believe is important for maintaining mental equilibrium.

A number of organic diseases—the pain of arthritis, difficulty in breathing, or pain due to heart or lung disease or other physical disabilities—can interfere with restful repose. Insomnia may be an indication of severe depression and is a prominent complaint among such patients. The symptom may have to be treated along with the disorder causing it. For a much larger number of us among the general population, however, insomnia is not the reflection of any deep underlying mental illness.

Treatment of the ordinary type of insomnia is multifaceted. Once a physician has ruled out any organic physical or severe mental illness, other contributing factors must be identified and controlled. A program of daily exercise may result in physical relaxation at bedtime. Caffeine-containing drinks consumed in the evening can interfere with our ability to fall asleep or stay asleep, and should be eliminated. Alcohol, although it induces sleep initially, may result in later restlessness that awakens us in the middle of the night. Certain medications might cause extensive mental stimulation and thus result in insomnia.

Occasionally a warm glass of milk may help. It was once thought that the amino acid L-tryptophan was the active ingredient in milk that induced sleep, but the amount in the ordinary glass of milk is too small to have any pharmacologic effect. Beneficial effects probably derive from some other component in the milk, or it's simply a psychological effect.

Drugs taken to induce sleep should be considered only as a last recourse. Although barbiturates have been largely replaced as sleep inducers by the less harmful **benzodiazapine** agents (including Valium and Dalmane), the latter are not without potentially serious side effects. Their elimination from the body may take several days, they can react with other medications, and a growing body of evidence is accumulating to indicate that they are addictive in many patients. Under no circumstances should they be taken on a daily basis except under the guidance of a properly qualified physician, especially if there is a demonstrated propensity or past history of drug dependency.

Self-help. Concern about lack of sleep can feed on itself, turning a minor, transient problem into a more serious one. It is important that we maintain a proper relaxed attitude toward this natural human process. "Catch-up sleep"—occasional longer periods of rest following a week or two of inadequate sleep time—is commonly employed by students and others who find this helpful in restoring normal wakefulness and vitality. Strategic napping, if possible, is another way of recharging our batteries and refreshing us for the hours ahead.

Finally, those awakening spontaneously in the middle of the night should not always resist this gift of time. Imagination and inventiveness can operate effectively at night without the day's normal distractions. Some of the world's great discoveries and artistic creations no doubt owe their origins just to such hours of creative restlessness. Such periods may even be therapeutic. Dr. James Minard, director of sleep-wake studies at the New Jersey Medical School, points out that while deprivation of REM sleep may aggravate manic illness, the effect seems to be just the opposite in depressed patients who, following deliberate curtailment of REM time, appear to have mood elevations and improved psychological functioning. Of course, it must be remembered that if insomnia is persistent and disabling, it may be an indication of some other problem and may require professional assistance.

Other Sleep Disorders

Other problems are connected to sleep, and deserve mention here. **Bed wetting** (enuresis) and **night terrors**—sudden attacks typically characterized by one's sitting up in bed and screaming—are childhood disorders, usually resolved after adolescence. In contrast to night terrors, in which we recall little of the content, the familiar adult **nightmare** is usually vividly remembered, especially immediately upon wakening. Nightmares are part of normal experience, but when particularly severe and/ or recurrent, some investigation may be in order. Certain drugs or an underlying mental illness may provoke severe nightmare activity.

Sleepwalking is not uncommon among children. About 15 percent of children experience at least one episode compared with the 2-to-4-percent rate among adults. When sleepwalking suddenly begins to occur in middle age or in the elderly, organic causes (such as a brain tumor) may be the inciting factor. **Talking in one's sleep** occurs commonly and requires no treatment.

Excessive sleepiness (hypersomnia) must be clearly distinguished from those people at the far end of the bell curve who sleep more than the average number of hours per night but are still within a normal range. Hypersomnia may represent part of the pattern of a depressive state or a side effect of some medication. Farther off the scale of normality is **narcolepsy,** a distressing syndrome typically characterized by the recurrent need for sleep. In early narcolepsy this may be the only waking symptom. Narcoleptics' reputation for sudden "sleep attacks" is probably due to **cataplexy**—a loss of muscle tension and weakness, with the patient collapsing to the floor in severe cases. The main danger in such patients is the risk of bodily harm to themselves and others, especially if they are driving automobiles or working in industrial settings at the time. The root cause of narcolepsy is a disturbance of the sleep-regulating area in the brain. The disorder can be clearly diagnosed by observation in a sleep laboratory, and can be helped by medication and strategic napping.

Sleep Apnea

Although included in this chapter, sleep apnea is a disorder firmly rooted in readily identified physical abnormalities of a man's anatomy, body weight, and cardiopulmonary function. The sleep manifestations of sleep apnea represent only the tip of the iceberg.

Patients who complain of this disorder are usually men between the ages of 40 and 60. They most often come to the attention of physicians because their mates notice their excessive snoring at night, followed by alarming periods when they stop breathing (apnea), then a resumption of even more snoring and perhaps choking sounds. On physical examination these patients are often, but not always, morbidly obese. They complain of excessive somnolence during the day and poor sleeping at night.

The same tissues in the back and sides of the throat that contribute to snoring can also be involved in the total obstruction that occurs intermittently with sleep apnea. As the person stops breathing, the oxygen levels in his blood drop and the carbon dioxide concentration climbs. Serious, even life-threatening cardiac arrhythmias occur. The diagnosis of sleep apnea can be established by overnight observation and recording in a sleep laboratory. In the obese, weight reduction is an important part of the treatment.

Some individuals with milder degrees of airway obstruction may need dental devices that are put in place at night to keep airways open. For more severe problems, currently the most widely prescribed form of therapy is **nasal continuous positive airway pressure** (NCPAP), in which a tight-fitting nasal mask connected by tubing to an air-flow generator is worn by the patient to ensure an adequately open airway and ventilation throughout the night.

Surgery to open the upper airway has been done with some success. In some severe cases a **tracheostomy** (a hole leading from the windpipe to the outside) may be required, at least temporarily, until other measures become effective.

DRUG AND ALCOHOL USE

Recent polls have shown that of all the domestic problems facing our society, drug addiction is of paramount concern to the American public. Alcohol and tobacco are not ordinarily thought of as drugs by most Americans, but their injudicious use accounts for more harm than that caused by all illicit substances combined.

What does "addiction" mean? Although this term is freely used among both laypersons and many health professionals, those dealing with such problems prefer to avoid it. They focus on either "drug use" or "drug dependency." Simply defined, *use* refers to the repeated use of a substance over a period of time, in such a way that it results in recurrent problems of social and mental functioning in the individual. *Dependence* may be psychological, connoting only adverse effects on mood following cessation of the drug, or physical, with clearly observed withdrawal symptoms (pain, sweating, nausea). Finally, *tolerance* refers to a person's need for increasing amounts of the substance in question to provide the desired effect. In alcoholics, for example, tolerance describes the ability to imbibe large amounts of alcohol before feeling its effects, quantities that would result in obvious inebriation among unaddicted individuals.

Whatever the terminology, it is eventually apparent to those in close contact with the drug-dependent person that there is a problem. Complicating the situation for those who would like to see the dependent person seek help is that often he denies the existence of any real problem.

Alcoholism

The social use of alcohol has traditionally been an integral part of many cultures, enhancing the enjoyment of food and easing social intercourse. Recent research indicates that the moderate consumption of alcohol (generally defined as no more than two drinks a day) may have a protective effect in terms of our resistance to the development of coronary heart disease, although this is still controversial.

In epidemiological terms, alcoholism is the major culprit in the death of almost 200,000 Americans annually. Money lost because of alcohol use, put at $117 billion in 1987, may reach approximately $150 billion per year by 1995. Half or more of the deaths resulting from traffic accidents, drowning, and homicides are related to alcohol, and nearly the same percentage of rapes and suicides are alcohol-related. About 10 percent of American men will have a problem with alcohol sometime during their lives. Alcoholism frequently exists as a component of many mental illnesses, but among the general population a genetic factor for alcoholism has been uncovered. Children of alcoholics are four times more likely to become alcoholic than children of nonalcoholics. Among identical twins it is twice as likely that both twins will be alcoholic as among fraternal twins. Among Native American tribes on reservations, where alcoholism is a major problem, studies have revealed an inability or diminished ability to metabolize alcohol in the liver.

Chronic alcoholism. The physical effects of chronic alcoholism are varied, and potentially affect many organs: the brain, peripheral nerves, the liver and gastrointestinal tract, the heart, the endocrine system, blood production, and the lungs. An increased susceptibility to cancer may also result from chronic alcohol use.

A number of acute withdrawal symptoms have been described among chronic alcoholics, ranging from the typical hangover to mild hallucinations to full-blown, life-threatening **delirium tremens** or hallucinations. At one time it was believed that poor nutrition, a frequent accompaniment to chronic alcoholism, was the cause of **cirrhosis of the liver** in alcoholics. It is now established that alcohol itself destroys liver cells. The loss of viable cells in the liver can result in liver failure. Cirrhosis, or scarring, can lead to obstruction to venous channels in the liver, with formation of **varices of the esophagus. Peptic ulcers** and **gastritis** (inflammation of the stomach lining) are also associated with alcohol.

In addition to effecting changes in the personality and destroying one's ability to operate normally at home and at work, alcoholism causes damage to the brain cells and can permanently affect the intellect. Damage to peripheral nerves from alcohol may result in pain, loss of sensation, and severe weakness.

Thirty years ago, no one commonly associated alcohol with heart disease. Today alcoholic heart disease is among the most common diagnoses made among cardiac patients in hospitals. Damage to the heart muscle may result in enlargement of the heart and eventual heart failure. An earlier effect of excessive alcohol intake may be irregularities of the heartbeat, typically occurring after a weekend or other time of more heavy drinking. Because of the association of those arrhythmias with such binging, this has been called the "holiday heart" syndrome, an early warning sign of what is to come unless sobriety intervenes.

Decreased resistance to lung and other infections is common among alcoholics. Cancer of the tongue, mouth, esophagus, and liver also are higher in alcoholics. Gonadal function is impaired. The litany of alcohol-related disorders can go on almost ad infinitum.

Acute alcoholism. Alcohol is a toxic substance. Excessive amounts, even when ingested by those without a long history of alcohol use, can result in coma and death. Even among chronic alcoholics, what might be considerd a moderate amount can result in death, especially during cold weather, when the dilation of blood vessels in the skin by the alcohol can cause severe drops in body temperature.

Treatment. It is important to deal with chronic alcoholism before it results in irreparable physical and mental harm. Various screening tests and standards have been devised to define and identify the alcoholic. In general they have included abnormal craving for the drug, blackouts, ability to tolerate large amounts of alcohol, and an inability to function at all without some alcohol because of tremulousness and other withdrawal symptoms. Both physicians and family have come to recognize the strong tendency for denial in such patients.

In the past, aversion therapy was one popular approach: The alcoholic was given a drug such as **disulfiram** (Antabuse), which produces extremely noxious effects when followed by alcohol. Some patients became seriously ill following this combination, however, and even a few deaths were reported, tempering the initial enthusiasm for this somewhat simplistic approach.

A more effective program involves a relatively intense regimen, either as an inpatient or an outpatient in a recognized facility dealing with such problems. Detoxification in the hospital is accomplished with the temporary assistance of drugs that ward off severe withdrawal symptoms. A concurrent program of abstinence is accompanied by psychiatric assistance.

Alcoholics Anonymous remains a valuable avenue of approach for many, although the spiritual orientation of the typical meeting has been alienating to some potential members. This has led to the establishment of some alternate AA chapters with a more secular orientation.

Although frequent failures in abstinence occur among alcoholics, the actual figures from reputable sources are not quite as discouraging as one might otherwise believe. One-year abstinence rates of 50 percent or greater are not unusual among many clinics.

What about "controlled drinking"? In 1976 some reports began to appear indicating that former alcoholics could resume moderate drinking without falling once again into the alcoholic abyss. The attractiveness of this idea—especially to alcoholics—still persists in some quarters. But long-term follow-up studies on the "successes" originally reported have almost invariably shown ultimate failure in most cases. Although controlled drinking may be applicable to a small number of borderline alcoholics, abstinence is the only solution for the great majority.

Marijuana

Marijuana is unquestionably the most commonly used of illicit drugs. For many years the major concern about marijuana use centered not on the effects of the drug itself, but rather on its role as providing social access to hard drugs such as cocaine and heroin. This "steppingstone" theory has some validity. Of those young men who have never used marijuana, only one percent will one day use cocaine or heroin. Of those who have been heavy users of marijuana (more than a thousand times), over two-thirds will eventually try cocaine and one-third heroin. Experimental use is common, however, especially among teenagers and young adults, and such use does not automatically condemn the user to later illicit drug use.

But as a greater number of studies on the effects of acute and chronic marijuana smoking have accumulated, confidence in the benign nature of this drug has diminished. Impairment of driving, slowed learning ability, and a falloff in the performance of skilled mental tasks have been shown repeatedly in studies of acute marijuana use. These effects can persist for hours. Marijuana use in some individuals produces panic or psychotic reactions.

The effects of chronic use are even more disturbing from a medical standpoint. Youthful marijuana smokers have often contended that at least their chosen weed was not as harmful as tobacco. However, the same changes in the lungs following tobacco smoking are seen with marijuana. Whether a propensity for lung cancer and heart disease follows marijuana use as it does tobacco use remains to be seen. For young people looking forward to parenthood, marijuana also has shown some troubling effects. In laboratory animals as well as humans, evidence of decreased sexual hormone production has been demonstrated. The use of marijuana (or cocaine) by pregnant women results in infants with low birth weight. Any potential contribution to this effect by the father's exhaled smoke being inhaled by the mother is unknown.

Cocaine

In the 1970s, cocaine rapidly became the drug of choice among many, especially the wealthy who could afford its high price tag. Because it did not require injection and its withdrawal symptoms were not yet recognized, cocaine was thought to be a relatively innocuous drug, especially when compared with heroin.

Although many can use cocaine only occasionally and not develop serious addiction, in many others it does lead to a pattern of compulsive use. It is in the powdered form, **cocaine hydrochloride,** that the drug is sniffed. When converted to "free base," it can be used intravenously but more often is smoked. It is as a smoke that an easily prepared and relatively inexpensive form of the base, **crack,** has come into wide use over the past five years. In this form, cocaine is much more rapidly addicting than by the nasal-sniffing route.

Cocaine can cause a sense of extreme euphoria, enormous energy, and sharpened mental acuity. With sniffing, this effect lasts an hour or more; with smoking, the high is achieved more rapidly and potently, but wears off within 20 minutes or so. The rapid decline in effect and the unpleasant sensations that the decline induces promote the repeated use of the drug at closer and closer intervals. Following such a binge, a three-phase pattern of abstinence follows: **crash, withdrawal,** and **extinction.**

The crash immediately following the loss of the drug effect can be compared to the hangover after an alcoholic bout. It is characterized by extreme exhaustion, often accompanied by anxiety and agitation. There is frequently a craving for sleep that is difficult to achieve, leading to the excessive use of hypnotics or opiates to obtain rest. Withdrawal symptoms—lack of energy and moroseness—follow the crash and persist (12 to 96 hours) with varying intensity, depending upon the previous pattern of drug use. Extinction refers to recurring episodes of craving for the drug in the days, weeks, or months following habitual use.

In contrast to marijuana, it is the acute physical effects of cocaine that are most alarming to the medical doctor, especially the effects on the brain and cardiovascular system. With or

without clotting of the coronary arteries, spasm may occur, causing occlusions and heart attacks indistinguishable clinically from
those occurring among coronary patients. Life-threatening cardiac arrthymias can occur. The marked rise in blood pressure
can cause bleeding into the brain, with resultant stroke damage,
especially in those with preexisting hypertension. In addition
to paralyzing strokes, severe generalized convulsions may follow cocaine ingestion, and marked elevations in body temperature have also been observed.

Contrary to popular mythology, sexual malfunction rather
than increased sexual performance and enjoyment is the norm
in both men and women users. Underlying psychological problems are often aggravated by cocaine use.

It is not known why sudden death can occur in those using
only relatively small amounts of cocaine for the first or second
time. Generalized convulsions, fatal cardiac arrhythmias, and
respiratory failure have all been implicated in such instances.
Some individuals may lack adequate amounts of the enzyme
necessary to metabolize cocaine; others may have an idiosyn-
cratic reaction to the drug, leading to extreme toxicity and death.

Treatment of acute cocaine intoxication is directed to reversing
any deleterious effects noted in the nervous and cardiovascular
systems. Long-term treatment involves individual and/or group
psychotherapy, with attention to environmental factors and behavior modification. Drugs such as **imipramine, desipramine,
lithium,** and others may play a role in halting the addiction.

Opioids (Heroin)

Although the term *opioid* refers to a wide variety of substances
that produce similar effects (**morphine, Demerol, Dilaudid,
methadone**), it is the intravenous or subcutaneous ("skin pop-
ping") use of heroin that represents the major problem with
this drug in the United States.

Physical dependency upon heroin is well recognized by the
public through fictional and media portrayals of addicts. Accidental overdosage can result in death due to severe respiratory
depression. It is the breaking of the skin barrier through contaminated needles and syringes, however, that results in consequences more severe—the transmission of fatal microbial

diseases such as AIDS. Immunological damage as the result of either the heroin or the vehicle with which it is diluted ("cut") is a probable factor in its potential for tissue damage, but is less well studied and understood.

Infection of heart valves by bacteria is a greatly feared complication of intravenous drug use. In one high-prevalance area, nearly one-third of all inpatient ultrasound studies of the heart are performed in addicts suspected of harboring such infections. Viral hepatitis is also relatively common among this patient group. Kidney failure (heroin nephropathy) is another serious complication, requiring chronic hemodialysis for the remainder of the patient's life.

Other Forms of Drug Use

The potentially harmful effects of sleeping pills have been discussed previously in the section on sleep disorders. In terms of other, more frankly illicit drugs, there are a variety of concoctions devised to remove us from, or "enhance," our senses. **Psychedelic drugs** such as LSD (lysergic acid), peyote, and mescaline were popular during the 1960s. Although these do not produce the physical dependence noted with heroin or cocaine, they can trigger acute psychotic episodes in the user. Another unpleasant effect may be "flashbacks"—spontaneous episodes of mental disturbance recurring up to many months following discontinuance of the drug.

PCP (phencyclidine) appeared on the streets in the late 1960s as the "peace pill," but later became better known as "angel dust." Because of the ease with which it can be synthesized, a cheap supply rapidly became available. It can be taken in a variety of ways, but it is usually sprinkled on marijuana and smoked. Although introduced as a surgical anesthetic by the pharmaceutical industry, PCP's popular desired effect is euphoria. A number of unpleasant and even dangerous side effects, including mania and convulsions, have been reported.

Amphetamines are well-recognized central nervous stimulants that at one time were frequently prescribed as part of many weight-reducing programs and have also been taken to maintain wakefulness. The effects of use and withdrawal are similar to those of cocaine, but usually less pronounced. As "speed," methamphetamine has had recurrent popularity. It has emerged in several urban areas in a new combination with mescaline known on the streets as **ecstasy.**

Of greater concern nationally and even internationally is a problem highlighted by the 1988 Olympics in Korea. This is the widespread use of **anabolic steroids,** which are male hormones or testosterone-type preparations. Not only has this type of substance penetrated the sphere of world-class athletes; it is used by many young American men. A 1988 nationwide study of male high school seniors revealed that nearly 7 percent had used anabolic steroids. One-fourth of these users, it turns out, were seeking improved physical appearance rather than enhanced athletic performance.

Although the long-term effects of this intentional disruption of the body's endocrinologic balance is unknown, there is ample cause for concern. In addition to their effects on muscle growth, steroids can change the salt composition of the body, affecting blood pressure. Although less frequently seen, long-term use can also cause liver cancer. In facing the problem of later possible effects of this form of drug use, medical investigators are haunted by the memory of another form of hormone administration and its disastrous aftermath: the use of **diethylstilbesterone** (DES), a female hormone that was found effective at one time in treating women with certain problems early in their pregnancies. In the early seventies it became apparent that in the daughters of such women there was an alarmingly high incidence of cancers of the female genital tract.

A final practical consideration for all those who believe that they can indulge in only casual or intermittent use of such illicit substances is the fact that spot testing for drug use is becoming increasingly common in every segment of business and industry. With some substances (PCP and marijuana, for example), urine samples will test positive even for several days or more following the use of such drugs. Thus even the truly nonaddicted individual may turn up as a marked man and face the risk of disciplinary action or even job loss.

Tobacco

The harmful effects of cigarette smoking in terms of coronary heart disease, lung disease, and cancer are well recognized.

A more recent problem in the area of tobacco involves the increased use of **smokeless tobacco** (snuff and chewing tobacco), especially among young males. Although this form of tobacco use avoids the effects of smoke inhalation upon the lungs, it still results in substantial absorption of nicotine, causing increases in blood pressure and heart rate as well as decreased blood flow to the skin. It may also aggravate peptic ulcer disease. Although such effects may not pose major threats to the young, the effects on dental hygiene are undeniable. An increased risk of cheek and gum cancer can affect all age groups.

For the vast majority of cigarette smokers, the question is not "Should I stop smoking?" but "How can I stop smoking?" Nicotine is a very addicting drug, and for many the habit is difficult to break. Yet there is ample evidence in the United States that major decreases in use have occurred among middle-aged men and especially among male physicians. A large part of the decrease in the incidence of coronary heart disease among American men observed in the last two decades has been attributed to cessation of their smoking habit.

The initial approach, in addition to individual counseling and education, is primarily one of self-management. If a smoker cannot stop "cold turkey," he should try to set up a timetable for reducing cigarette consumption, followed by complete cessation. It's preferable to substitute other oral substances (low-calorie candy, gum) to gratify the oral craving. (Incidentally, the fear of significant weight gain due to increased appetite following abstinence has been greatly exaggerated, as shown by several recent studies.) To reduce temptation, it's best to avoid situations where smoking is likely to occur, and not to get discouraged by occasional lapses.

Therapists are available who use contingency management and aversion therapy. The first uses self-determined rewards and punishments for success or failure. Aversion therapy, which can range from deliberate exposure to noxious amounts of smoke to electroconvulsive therapy, requires professional participation.

Nicotine gum (and more recently, preliminary trials of nicotine-containing skin patches) has been used with varying success. Although it may alleviate craving, the systemic effects of nicotine may be harmful to middle-aged and older patients with heart and other types of chronic disease. Other drug treatment has been tried. **Clonidine,** a drug used for lowering blood pressure, and which has some sedative effects on the brain, has been used to reduce the craving for nicotine during acute withdrawal. Hypnosis and acupuncture have had limited success.

What about filter cigarettes? Perhaps most smokers today are using some form of filter. Although this may result in a lower cancer mortality, switching to filters does not seem to lower the risk for coronary heart disease.

Another possibility is to switch to a pipe or cigar. The incidence of coronary heart disease, lung disease, and lung cancer may be slightly higher for cigar and pipe smokers than for nonsmokers, but this is of questionable statistical significance. For light smokers of cigars (less than six a day) or pipes (less than ten pipefuls daily), there is probably no difference in the above diseases when compared with the nonsmoking population. The one medical area is which there is a clear-cut risk from pipe and cigar smoking involves cancer of the mouth cavity, lip (in pipe smokers), tongue, and larynx. As with cigarette smokers, there is also an increased risk of esophageal cancer. When one considers that cancer accounts for about 20 percent of all deaths in the United States, that cancers of the oral cavity constitute only 5 percent of these, and that such cancers are often amenable to early detection and cure, the option for switching to pipes or cigars—if in moderation—may seem a desirable one. Unfortunately, though, blood studies in former cigarette smokers who have switched to these other modes indicate that inhalation continues despite the change in tobacco product. Thus any benefits that might otherwise be gained are not worth the effort.

One spur to quitting the cigarette habit is the realization that although previous lung damage from smoke cannot be reversed, its progression can be halted. Furthermore, risk of lung and other cancers can be markedly reduced. Finally, the threefold risk of coronary heart disease in the pack-a-day smoker can be cut in half with a year of stopping, and the increased risk of coronary heart disease can be eliminated completely after ten years of abstinence.

PSYCHOTHERAPY

To many men, psychotherapy means the analytic couch presided over by a psychiatrist who follows strict Freudian principles and practices. Although this intensive, prolonged type of treatment is still employed, the number of patients in need of psychiatric treatment that are being treated this way represents a distinct minority. For most cases, classical psychoanalysis takes too long, is too expensive, and, in current health-care terminology, is not cost-effective.

Today, various types of health professionals administer psychotherapy. Where drugs must be used, a psychiatrist, alone among such therapists, can write the requisite prescriptions because a psychiatrist must be an M.D. In other settings, psychologists or psychiatric social workers may deal with cases. Such individuals usually have at least master's degrees or, frequently, Ph.D.'s in psychology.

A shorter form of treatment that utilizes psychodynamic principles similar to those of classical psychoanalysis is called **psychoanalytic therapy**. In this form of treatment the focus is on resolving current problems rather than delving back into childhood experiences and psychic trauma. A relatively rapid, supportive alliance with the psychotherapist is the goal, and the patient can, with some insight, be relieved of his symptoms and begin to cope with life more effectively.

Because of the increasing pressures of patient load and time and cost constraints, even shorter courses of psychotherapy are being attempted, usually lasting no more than a dozen sessions or so and not exceeding three or four months in duration. A spinoff of this trend is **crisis intervention** for particularly acute episodes of psychological disturbance. It consists of immediate psychiatric treatment of as few as one or two interviews or up to a month or two of treatment. Many crisis-intervention centers are located within or adjacent to hospital emergency rooms where, in psychiatric terms, they operate analogously to medical or surgical emergency services in the provision of prompt and effective care.

Under the direction of a skilled psychotherapist, **group therapy,** on either an inpatent or outpatient basis, has proved helpful for certain types of problems. It may or may not be combined with individual psychotherapy. Drug users, prisoners, veterans, and others have participated actively in such programs. **Psychodrama,** in which patients actually act out their problem situations, under the guidance of a counselor, might be considered an offshoot of group therapy. **Self-help** groups (those operating without the supervision of a trained psychotherapist) also have a role, as clearly demonstrated by Alcoholics Anonymous and other groups.

Family therapy is indicated in the treatment of some psychiatric ailments. In anorexia nervosa, for example, the participation of all family members is usually considered an essential element of treatment.

Behavior therapy is used in an increasingly wide variety of conditions. One component of this approach is desensitization to fear-inducing circumstances (e.g., phobias such as agoraphobia). **Aversion therapy,** using noxious stimulants to discourage undesired behavior, is also included under this therapeutic mantle.

Hypnosis has been utilized to bring unconscious memories to consciousness and to attempt to alter behavior patterns through posthypnotic suggestion. It is not currently a prominent modality in psychiatry. Long-term lack of effectiveness is probably the reason for the diminished interest in this approach.

Of greater growing importance than hypnosis is the use of **cognitive therapy.** The theoretical basis for this approach is that some patients' major problem is an inability to perceive reality; it is this that leads to their inappropriate behavior and psychological distress. The role of the psychiatrist here is first to reveal to the patient the errors of his perception, and then to help him adopt behavior more consonant with reality. Such treatment is usually intense and individualized and relies greatly on the psychiatrist's active participation, in contrast to the more passive receptive role of the psychotherapist in the psychoanalytic setting.

Drugs and Psychotherapy

The second half of the twentieth century has been remarkable for the development of effective drug therapy, in psychiatry no less than in other branches of medicine. The introduction of **chlorpromazine** (Thorazine) in the mid-1950s revolutionized the management of previously uncontrollable psychotic inpatients. At about the same time, lithium became available for the treatment of manic depression.

Today a wide spectrum of drugs that either inhibit excessive brain activity or relieve depressive manifestations of mental illness are part of the basic pharmacologic tools used by the practicing psychiatrist. These drugs are all potent, capable in varying degrees of inducing mild to severe side effects, and require the supervision of a knowledgeable psychiatrist in the course of their administration. In almost all cases some psychotherapy should also be included as part of the treatment plan.

7

Care of the Skin and Hair

THE SKIN

Although few people think of it as such, the skin constitutes
the largest organ of the body. It's also the one that first attracts
attention when something goes awry. With the possible exception of male-pattern baldness, none of the disorders common
to the skin can be described as peculiar to men. But good,
healthy skin is essential to a man's physical and psychological
well-being; he also should be alert to those diseases that first
manifest themselves as skin disorders.

How the Skin Functions

The skin is made up of three layers: The most superficial is
called the **epidermis,** under this is the **dermis,** and the deepest
layer is fatty **subcutaneous tissue.**

The epidermis is paper-thin, but it contains many layers of
cells. New cells are constantly produced from the deepest portion of the epidermis, and push up to the surface to replace

older cells that have become flattened, dried out, and eventually sloughed off. This process is called **keratinization,** and cells involved in this constant regeneration constitute about 95 percent of those in the epidermis. Also located in this layer of the skin are cells called **melanocytes.** These contain various amounts of pigment and account for most of the color of our skin. Sunlight stimulates greater production of pigment within these cells and produces the tanning effect after exposure. Hair and nails are also considered part of the epidermis.

The dermis is a more substantial skin layer than the epidermis, and is more complex. It contains nerve fibers and some muscle cells. Imbedded in the dermis are sweat glands that help to dissipate heat through the evaporation of their secretions. There are also hair follicles and sebaceous glands that secrete an oily material, **sebum,** that migrates to the surface of the skin along the hair shaft. Blood vessels running through the dermis also help to preserve body heat (when they constrict) or dissipate it (when they dilate). They also affect our complexion, as observed when we blanch or blush.

The subcutaneous tissue, deep in the dermis, varies in distribution and depth over the body, with easily appreciated differences between the two sexes. It protects, cushions against hard contacts, serves as an insulator, and stores caloric energy within its fat cells.

One of the most important of skin functions is to shelter the underlying structures of the body from chemical or other harmful substances encountered in the environment. The bodily fluids necessary for normal function are kept intact beneath its protective mantle. Temperature regulation, already touched upon, is another vital role of the skin. The skin is also an essential component of our physical appearance, and as such it represents an important psychological element of our self-image.

DISORDERS OF THE SKIN

Rashes

Although many systemic diseases (those affecting many areas of the body) can have skin manifestations as part of the picture, in other diseases the problem is limited to the skin.

With **dermatitis** or skin inflammation, there is a reddening of the skin, frequently accompanied by itching and possible localized swelling or blisters.

Dermatitis can be caused by irritating substances or as a result of allergy. In the first category are many chemicals. Mechanical factors, such as the rubbing of skin surfaces together, or contact of skin with rough clothing, can result in rashes. Allergic rashes can result from a variety of foods, and the number of drugs that may result in allergic skin rashes are legion. Commonly used prescriptions involve penicillin and related antibiotics, sulfa drugs, **griseofulvin** (used for fungal infections), tetracycline, **diphenylhydantoin** (Dilantin), antihistamines, barbiturates, and **phenothiazines.**

Any rash that appears following ingestion of a drug should raise the question of a possible link. The fact that the drug has previously been taken without ill effect does not exclude the possibility of rash, since allergic reactions to a drug may not occur until the drug has been taken multiple times in the past.

The most important aspect of treating drug- or food-related skin allergy is recognition of the cause and elimination of the offending agent.

Contact dermatitis is a form of skin reaction caused by specific areas of the body coming into contact with an inciting substance. The cause may be allergy or direct chemical or physical irritation. Some strong soaps or detergents can affect the hands in this way. Metal on a bracelet or ring may cause a rash in the underlying skin area. Poison oak and poison ivy also represent forms of contact dermatitis.

In addition to avoiding substances and objects that cause such skin reactions, the itching and inflammation can be reduced by applying the appropriately prescribed salves, most commonly topical cortisone-like or steroid skin creams or ointments, to be applied until the condition resolves itself.

Urticaria, or hives, is a rather acute form of allergic skin reaction characterized by the sudden apppearance of itchy welts over the body that usually resolve spontaneously over a few days, or more quickly if treated with antihistamines.

Intertrigo is a form of skin irritation caused by the continuous rubbing together of two skin surfaces. In men, this problem is usually more common with obesity and may involve the armpits, the groin, or the inner thighs, especially in hot weather. Keep such areas dry with the use of powders following showers, and wear boxer shorts rather than tight briefs. At night, use the minimum number of blankets to prevent overheating and sweating. Eliminating pajama bottoms or sleeping completely in the nude also may prove beneficial. Occasionally, intertrigo may become complicated by bacterial or fungal infection, and your doctor can prescribe the appropriate topical treatment.

Recurrent or persistent skin rashes, unrelated to specific identifiable causes, usually fall into the category of atopic or other forms of chronic dermatitis of uncertain cause. These irritations may require the continued and expert management of a dermatologist over the long term.

Acne

Acne is a condition that strikes adolescents; over three-quarters of maturing males experience some degree of acne, with the peak prevalence at age 17. The skin changes that provoke acne usually diminish by young adulthood, although problems may persist in some men. Occasionally the condition becomes very extensive or severe, and complications may arise.

Symptoms. As described before, sebaceous glands within the dermis layer of skin produce an oily material, sebum, that migrates up to the surface via the hair shaft in order to lubricate the skin. In acne the passage becomes obstructed because of increased keratinization of the most superficial layers of the skin. The process is most marked during adolescence, because at this time increasing amounts of male hormones (androgens) are produced, which stimulate the activity of the sebaceous glands.

The main visible effect of this process is called the **comedone,** or, in popular terms, a pimple or "zit." The closed comedone (whitehead) occurs when the impacted sebum is trapped below the surface in barely visible small swellings. Blackheads develop when the sebum is combined with skin pigments.

In more severe forms of acne, the blocked sebum collects in cysts, which may rupture, irritating and inflaming the skin. Secondary infection with bacteria and other microorganisms can exacerbate the process. Finally, scarring of the skin in varying degrees may be the end result. The lesions of acne are usually confined to the face and neck, although in more severe cases the shoulders, chest, and upper back may also become involved.

Although androgens play an important role in acne, a more decisive cause is heredity. Where one or both parents had problems with acne in their youth or beyond, their offspring are much more likely to develop it than are those whose parents had minimal problems in this regard.

Treatment. There are many approaches to the treatment of acne, depending upon the extent of the problem. Most people can manage a case of mild acne on their own with frequent and thorough skin cleansing (two to three times a day), taking care not to irritate the skin by too-vigorous rubbing. Shampooing the hair two to three times weekly will also help to decrease the amount of oil on the skin.

When topical medication is required for better control, preparations containing **benzoyl peroxide** are recommended. This chemical is antibacterial in its action. It also helps to eliminate comedones and excessive superficial skin. Available in prescription form or over-the-counter, it is prepared in different strengths and in various forms: as a lotion (Benzoyl, Oxy-5, Persadox, Vanoxide); as a cream (Clearasil, Cuticura, Acne-aid); and as a gel (Benzac, Benzagel, Desquam-X, PanOxyl, Persa-Gel). Some may note a mild redness and scaling of the skin, which may occur during the first week or two of use. The liquid and cream formulations tend to be less irritating than the gel forms of the drug, although the gel forms may be more effective.

For more severe or resistant acne, sufferers should seek the help of a dermatologist. For some people, a derivative of vitamin A, **Accutane**, may be prescribed in oral form. This agent is a potent and effective drug for the treatment of cystic acne, but it is reserved for only the most intractable cases because of its many possible side effects. Among these are dry skin, chapped lips, and nosebleeds; more serious complications include liver function abnormalities, headaches, and bone problems. But the most serious side effect is the very real possibility of birth defects in children whose mothers took the drug when pregnant. For this reason it is mandatory that women use some form of birth control when taking the drug. Effective contraception must be used for at least one month before the start of Accutane therapy, during therapy, and for one month after the therapy has ended.

Other treatments for severe acne include the use of oral antibiotics and corticosteroids.

Two final notes on acne treatment: Everyone has a tendency to pick or squeeze unsightly pimples and blackheads. This can result in further inflammation and scarring. Finally, the effect of diet on acne, although often hotly discussed in the past, does not seem to have any firm scientific foundation. An overemphasis on "proper" and "improper" foods, especially by parents, can only add to the emotional strains already imposed by the problem itself.

Scarring. The end result of long-standing and severe acne may be extensive and unsightly scarring of the skin. Once the inflammatory aspects have subsided, a process called **dermabrasion** may be attempted by your dermatologist to restore a more normal appearance of the skin surface. This procedure involves planing down the skin surface with a high-speed wire brush. It should be done only by those experienced in the technique. Success is not really predictable, with reported improvement (as perceived by patients) ranging from 30 to 75 percent. Infection, loss or increase of skin pigmentation, and new scarring as a result of the procedure itself are occasional complications.

An alternative to dermabrasion is **collagen implantation.** In this technique, highly purified collagen, a protein obtained from cattle, is injected under the pitted areas to elevate them to the same level as the surrounding normal skin. This requires between two and six injections at two-to-four-week intervals until the desired result is obtained. To maintain this, subsequent injections must be administered at intervals ranging from six months to two years. About 3 percent of the population will have an allergy to the protein, so the dermatologist will perform a skin test with the collagen prior to treatment. Similarly, people with arthritis and other connective-tissue diseases are not suitable candidates for collagen because the foreign protein might aggravate their condition. More recently, silicone injections, which do not require repeated treatment, have been available as an alternative approach.

Psoriasis

Psoriasis affects about 1 to 2 percent of the white population and includes both men and women. Although it can begin at any age, it usually starts in the twenties. There is an inherited tendency for development of the disease, with about one-third of those affected reporting a family history of psoriasis. It is not contagious, but it is not curable. Although psoriasis can often be controlled with proper medication, recurrences are common and unpredictable.

Symptoms. The basic problem in psoriasis is an accentuation of the normal process of skin renewal. As superficial layers of dead skin are shed with the normal wear and tear of living, their loss is replaced by the production of new skin cells. In psoriasis this process in certain areas of the skin is excessive, resulting in the appearance of the typical reddened plaque with its margins distinct from the surrounding normal skin. Silvery white scales, representing shed skin, often cover the psoriatic plaque.

Common locations of the plaques are the elbows and knees, although the scalp may frequently be included. Occasionally the armpits, groin, and nail beds are also involved. Some individuals, in addition to the skin manifestations, develop an arthritis that is very similar in symptoms and appearance to rheumatoid arthritis.

Itching is not a prominent feature in psoriasis. An exception to this may be when the scalp is involved, and the disease may be confused with **seborrheic dermatitis** (severe dandruff). The skin lesions of psoriasis tend to get better in the summer, when they are exposed to sunlight, although there are some individuals in whom just the opposite seems to be the case.

Treatment. The treatment of psoriasis depends upon both the extent of the skin problem and the psychosocial setting in which it occurs. When large areas of the body surface are involved, there is usually no question about the need for an aggressive approach to managing it. At other times, when only small areas are affected, the approach will vary depending upon the sufferer. An elderly male with only two or three small patches of skin involved may shrug it off as only one more minor burden of growing older. A young, sexually active person, concerned about his appearance and attractiveness, may find the same lesions devastating.

Inasmuch as there is no real cure for psoriasis, it is understandable that a number of remedies have been developed over the years in attempts to find the most effective means of reducing the extent and impact of the disorder. Fortunately, many fairly safe drugs are obtainable either over-the-counter or by prescription, and they are effective in most people. More-potent, potentially harmful agents are reserved for only those with the most resistant and extensive types of the disease.

Coal-tar preparations, in various formulations, have been used in psoriasis for over a hundred years. Coal tar consists of many compounds, and why it works in psoriasis is not really understood, but it is effective. A problem with older preparations of coal tar was that they were smelly and messy to use. Newer formulations are more esthetically acceptable but may not work quite as well. Coal-tar medications are applied to affected areas for several hours—usually overnight—and then cleaned off. Redness is reduced and scaling diminished through a reduction in skin overproduction in the patches treated.

Some examples of coal-tar preparations include Aqua-Tar Gel, Doak Tar Lotion, Estar Gel, Bainetar, and Tarbonis cream. Coal tar can also be obtained in combination with **allantoin,** a skin-softening agent (Psorex, Tegrin), or with **salicylic acid,** perhaps an even more reliable softening agent, to help in the removal of scales.

As with many skin conditions, **steroids** have replaced many of the older remedies that were often prescribed in the past. Steroid creams, ointments, or lotions vary in strength and are often potent in their anti-inflammatory effect without the risk of complications when applied to the skin. **Triamcinolone** (Aristocort, Kenalog), in the form of a .5-percent cream or ointment, is a common formulation employed. More-potent steroids are acceptable alternatives when this does not suffice. Some dermatologists prefer to inject small amounts of steroid just under the affected skin patches for more-rapid and perhaps more-lasting responses.

Taking steroids by mouth is rarely if ever advised in psoriasis because of the many potentially severe side effects that may occur.

Anthralin is a topical preparation that has been found effective in the treatment of very thick, stubborn psoriasis plaques that have proved unresponsive to other topical agents. It is usually applied as an overnight preparation. It may be irritating to the skin and cause stinging. For this reason it is not employed as a first choice or when inflammation is a prominent feature of the plaques to be treated. For the same reason, short-term applications (for example, a half hour at a time) may be substituted for overnight treatment.

For those with large areas of psoriasis, involving 50 percent of the body surface or more, the beneficial effects of **ultraviolet light** have been recognized for many years. In the 1920s the **Goeckerman regimen** was introduced and is still a recognized effective treatment. It involves the application of coal tar followed by exposure to artificially produced ultraviolet light or even sunlight itself.

More recently, an alternative ultraviolet treatment has been employed: **PUVA** (psoralen ultraviolet A). This utilizes a specific range of ultraviolet light in combination with **psoralen,** an agent that enhances skin sensitivity to ultraviolet light. The treatment appears to be highly effective, with about a 90-percent success rate reported. However, the course of therapy is both expensive and time-consuming, involving visits to the dermatologist's "light box" two to three times a week for a total of eight to 12 weeks to complete a course of treatment. Concerns have been expressed about all this ultraviolet light aging the skin and, more important, the possibility that it could induce skin cancer. These concerns have tempered enthusiasm for an otherwise effective approach to extensive psoriasis. (Long-term observations on patients who have undergone the Goeckerman treatment, incidentally, have not so far demonstrated an increased risk of skin cancer.)

Other psoriasis treatments are usually reserved as last-ditch attempts to deal exclusively with the most recalcitrant and severe forms of the disease. One approach involves the low-dose use of an anticancer drug, methotrexate, to suppress the production of skin cells. Newer treatments, not completely accepted and still undergoing evaluation, include the use of **vitamin A** derivatives (retinoids) and **vitamin D** and its metabolite, calcipotriol.

Skin Cancer

Skin cancers are among the most common malignancies that occur in men and women. In the United States each year, more than 500,000 individuals will develop some form of skin cancer. Skin cancer will eventually affect 40 to 50 percent of all those living to age 65 or beyond. The other side of the coin is that skin cancer is often curable and, most important, preventable.

Fair-skinned whites are most suceptible to skin cancers. The incidence of skin cancer among blacks is only 1 to 2 percent of that in whites; among Hispanics the incidence is about 12 percent that of whites. Men are twice as prone as women to develop skin cancer, and each individual's risk is related to the amount of exposure to the sun's rays or other ultraviolet light.

The most common skin cancers for which we are at risk are basal cell carcinomas (accounting for about 80 percent of the total), squamous cell carcinomas, and malignant melanomas. Malignant melanomas arise from the pigment-bearing cells of the skin and are of the most concern because of their relatively poor prognosis compared to other skin cancers. Approximately 20 percent of all those who develop malignant melanoma will ultimately die of the disease.

Unfortunately, all varieties of skin cancer seem to be on the increase. The key to reversing this trend is early recognition as well as prevention.

Basal cell carcinomas. The most commonly occurring kind of skin cancers, these begin on exposed areas of the skin—the face, hands, and forearms. The incidence is usually greatest after the age of 40; the lesions appear most frequently on eyelids, nose, forehead, or around the ears. Their appearance is typically that of a raised, hard, red or pearly gray elevation in the skin. Often the center is broken down, forming an ulcer or sore that fails to heal. This last aspect is an important clue that the lesion is something more than just a passing inflammation or injury to the skin.

Squamous cell carcinomas. These often arise from **actinic keratoses,** which are raised collections of scales in skin areas frequently exposed to the sun and wind over a long period. Like the basal cell carcinomas, they occur predominantly among the aging population. Squamous cell cancer is crusty in nature, tends to break down, and, like basal cell cancers, fails to heal over a period of several weeks or longer. While squamous cell cancers are much less common than basal cell cancers (about 20 percent of the total number of skin cancers), they tend to be more invasive and account for three-quarters of all skin cancer deaths after malignant melanomas.

Although a doctor may suspect that both of these types of skin lesions are cancerous, confirmation requires removal of the entire lesion (if it is small) or a portion of it for biopsy, so that a definitive microscopic diagnosis can be made. Skin cancers are classified by physicians on the basis of how deep within the skin they have penetrated, and whether or not they have spread to the local lymph nodes or beyond. The extent of spread will determine the prognosis.

A variety of treatments are available for the management of these two kinds of common skin cancers: topical application of anticancer drugs; surgery; and X-ray therapy (radiotherapy).

The cure rate for basal cell carcinomas is excellent (90 to 95 percent) and approaches 100 percent when the lesions are recognized early and treated promptly. This is especially true of those that are small, i.e., less than a centimeter (a little less than a half-inch) in diameter. Results of treatment are almost as good for squamous cell cancers, with cures generally in the 75-to-80-percent range with localized lesions. These results cannot be achieved when such cancers are neglected and allowed to grow or spread, so early diagnosis and therapy are mandatory.

Malignant melanomas. These differ from other skin cancers in several respects. Although the incidence peaks after the age of 50, these tumors also show a greater tendency than the others to appear at younger ages. They may appear as early as the twenties or thirties, with the incidence rising sharply into the forties and sixties. Although melanomas often appear on the exposed areas of the skin, they have a slightly greater tendency than the other skin cancers to appear on the trunk, thighs, and other areas of the body not ordinarily exposed to the sun.

The recognition of malignant melanoma by its appearance alone can be more difficult. The typical appearance can vary. Most often the skin lesions are described as "disorderly" with blurred margins and differing coloration within the perimeter— light and dark areas intermingling. They can also appear as uniformly blue-black or brownish.

Successful treatment here depends upon early diagnosis, because melanoma has a greater tendency to spread both locally and to distant parts of the body. The treatment is essentially surgical, since radiotherapy and chemotherapy have not been shown to be very effective. When the melanoma is superficial, surgical excision can result in five-to-ten-year survival rates of 95 percent or even greater. When the deeper layers of the skin have been penetrated, and especially when local lymph nodes are involved, the survival rates fall off sharply to about 30 to 50 percent. The outlook is most ominous when distant spread has occurred.

Prevention. The following are some personal guidelines regarding skin cancer:

- Avoid excessive exposure to sunlight. Use appropriate sunscreens and avoid the sun's rays from 11 A.M. to 3:00 P.M., when they are the most powerful.
- Be suspicious of any sores that fail to heal promptly, especially those in areas of the skin generally exposed to the sun. Have your personal doctor or a dermatologist check any suspicious moles, especially if they seem to be changing or growing larger.
- Seek professional help early, should you have any suspicion of a skin cancer.
- Do not resist excision or biopsy of suspicious lesions. Even expert dermatologists can be fooled by appearance alone. The dictum, "When in doubt, cut it out," is often the wisest to follow if skin cancers are to be managed successfully. Small bits of tissue, removed without leaving any cosmetic defect, can aid diagnosis one way or the other and prove critical for your best future interests.

ROUTINE CARE OF THE SKIN

Skin characteristics vary considerably from one person to another, with differences in color, texture, smoothness, hair distribution, and other qualities. In terms of routine skin care, however, there are three categories of skin—dry, normal, and oily—the category assignment depending upon the amount of material secreted by the sebaceous glands within the dermis.

Because skin problems often involve too much or too little oil, proper care must take this factor into account. If you have **dry skin,** excessive washing can further deplete natural oils and aggravate the condition. For this reason, avoid frequent showering or bathing in the colder months. Local washing with a sponge or cloth in certain areas (armpits, groin, feet) is preferable.

When you do bathe, use a bathtub rather than a shower, since showering is more likely to wash away precious body oils. Furthermore, immersion in a bath for 15 minutes or more can help to restore moisture to an overly dry skin. Following bathing, use moisturizing creams or lotions that will help hold in body moisture and prevent the flaking, cracking, and itching of dried-out skin. Use mild soaps and nonalkaline shampoos.

Low humidity in our homes, especially during the winter months, can often aggravate a dry skin condition. Heating systems that circulate hot air are particularly likely to result in suboptimal humidity. Humidifiers, raising the humidity to 30 or 35 percent, may assist greatly in the management of dry skin during such times of the year.

If you have **oily skin,** just the opposite rules apply. Frequent showering and hair shampooing with mild soaps and shampoos will reduce the oiliness and improve your skin's appearance.

Regardless of basic skin quality, it is now strongly recognized that important skin problems are related to exposure to excessive amounts of sunlight. The worst consequence of too much sun is not sunburn; it is skin cancer, the most common of all human malignancies.

Avoid the sun. It is the ultraviolet rays of the sun that predispose you to skin cancer, and these should be avoided as much as possible. The most intense of these rays occur between

11:00 A.M. and 3:00 P.M. Avoid outdoor activity during this part of the day to minimize exposure to these harmful rays.

Keeping parts of the body covered is another tactic, though not completely protective. About 20 percent of ultraviolet waves penetrate typical, loosely knit summer wear and reach the skin. The use of hats is advisable, especially for those with sparse hair. Seeking out shady areas is preferable to sitting exposed to direct sunlight, but radiation from bright reflective surfaces (beach sand, snow, or pavement) may easily reach you in the shade. Cloudy days offer little respite; as much as 70 to 80 percent of ultraviolet radiation from the sun may reach ground level even on days that are hazy or overcast.

Agents that protect against the harmful rays of the sun play a major role in skin protection. These are of two major types: sun blockers and sunscreens. A typical sun blocker is zinc oxide ointment, a thick white paste that is often applied to areas of the face particularly prone to excessive exposure—the lips, nose, or forehead. Sun blockers work by deflecting ultraviolet radiation.

Sunscreens, usually applied to larger areas over the surface of the body, absorb, reflect, or scatter ultraviolet radiation and can be obtained in various numerical strengths, each higher number connoting a greater degree of protection. Ratings vary from as low as 2, providing minimal protection, to 10, 15, or 25. The essential ingredient in many of these preparations is **PABA** (para-aminobenzoic acid) or one of its derivatives.

THE HAIR

Hair growth in animals and humans is cyclic. Fortunately for us, though, human hair growth is also asynchronous, which means that each scalp hair is growing or has discontinued its growth phase independently of its neighboring hairs. Otherwise we would shed all our hair periodically, as some animals do when they undergo a seasonal molt.

Hair Loss

However you look at it, for most men, losing one's hair is one of the most distressing aspects of growing older. More than two-thirds of all normal men will be affected in various degrees, usually in their thirties or forties, though signs of balding may be detected in some men as early as their twenties.

The development of male baldness follows a typical pattern. There is temporal hair loss, causing a receding hairline along the sides of the forehead and resulting in what has been called the "widow's peak" pattern. There is also thinning of hair on the crown, eventually causing a bald spot. In more severe baldness the receding hairline and the expanding bald spot merge, leaving only a ring of hair remaining around the sides and back of the head.

For those readers young enough to be in doubt about their own future prospects in the hair department, a look at their fathers and the family photograph album will provide important clues. Hair patterns are determined genetically. If grandfathers on both sides of the family tree had bald pates in their final years, it is likely that you will follow suit. If such is the case, what are your options to forestall or possibly reverse your pre-ordained hair loss?

Minoxidil (Rogaine). In the late 1970s, doctors were using a relatively new, potent anti-hypertensive drug for patients whose elevated blood pressure would not respond to the usually effective agents. Early on, a disturbing effect of the drug in question, minoxidil, was noted, especially in women: It caused unwanted hair growth. It did not take much imagination to envision putting this to a beneficial use: Put the drug in some kind of topical form that could be applied to the balding heads of men. Upjohn wasted no time in developing just such a preparation (Rogaine), which began to undergo clinical testing in 1983. What has been learned so far about its effectiveness and safety?

It appears that the major effect of minoxidil is the prevention of future hair loss rather than the restoration of hair that has already disappeared. In the latter case there is some true objective benefit, but it is hardly hair-raising in its magnitude. For example, the average normal density of scalp hair in the male is about 500 follicles per square centimeter. In one study of bald spots subjected to minoxidil over a year's time, there were an average of 31 new follicles per square centimeter—a truly positive effect, but with a resultant hair production only 6 percent of normal. In a similar study there was almost a threefold increase in hair follicles after minoxidil: from 29 to 83 follicles per square centimeter. But again, the success represented only 17 percent of what would normally be there. Furthermore, the new hairs that do sprout include, among sturdy, thick, dark hair shafts, a number of lesser structures that are technically hair but could also be described by a less kind observer as "fuzz."

There are undoubtedly those, probably in the range of 20 to 30 percent, who consider the treatment a success. And fortunately, for those who elect to try topical minoxidil, there are few contraindications (usually chronic inflammatory conditions in the scalp) and only minor side effects. About 3 percent of those using this treatment complain of dryness and itching of the scalp, probably related to the effects of the alcohol vehicle containing the minoxidil rather than the active agent itself.

Now for the bad news: It takes a minimum of four months for an effect to be noticed, and the minoxidil must be continued indefinitely; minoxidil is a *treatment* for baldness, not a cure. It costs between $50 and $85 for a month's supply, plus the cost of visits to the dermatologist's office. Will your insurance cover any of the cost? Probably not.

However modest the effect of minoxidil on baldness, and despite the high cost of treatment, minoxidil is a far cry from the kind of "snake oil" preparations that have been touted for the treatment of male baldness in the past, some of which continue to be widely promoted. It is the first agent approved officially by the Food and Drug Administration for this purpose, and, most important, it probably represents only the first of a number of similar preparations that will be available in the future from the laboratories of enterprising pharmaceutical corporations.

Other options. Toupees of vastly varying quality have been a staple resource for the balding man for centuries. But with the progression of surgical knowledge and techniques, **hair transplantation** has emerged as an alternative cover for barren patches.

The procedure involves the removal of tiny plugs of hair-growing skin at the back and sides of the head, scalp areas almost invariably unaffected by baldness. These are transplanted to bare areas of the scalp where they are needed. For optimal effectiveness, only small plugs are removed (8 to 15 follicles per plug), and only about 30 plugs at a time every month or so until the desired result is obtained. Because it must be done so gradually, the process is prolonged, somewhat tedious, and certainly labor-intensive. As a result, it is also expensive. It also involves short-term minor pain and numbness over the areas of surgery, but eventually this fades.

Is it all worth it? Close observation of others who have undergone this treatment will reveal, even to the nonexpert, that the results can vary markedly. In some men the evidence of hair transplantation is almost unnoticeable and the cosmetic effect excellent. In others it looks as if a miniaturized hairy minefield has exploded. An alternative to multiple small skin grafts is the use of large segments or pedicles of scalp with hair relocated surgically to balding areas, but this is a more radical approach.

Suitability for transplants may vary from one balding individual to another. Skills at performing this procedure can also vary widely among dermatologists. If you have decided to undergo this treatment, one wise recommendation is that you aak a dermatologist who does *not* perform transplants to recommend a good one who does. Before undergoing this prolonged and expensive course of treatment, it might also be wise to review a gallery of before-and-after photographs of previous patients in order to achieve a realistic impression of what you yourself might expect as the final result.

Dandruff

Dandruff is a mild form of seborrheic dermatitis, a condition in which there is excessive scaling of the skin, especially on the scalp. This condition can usually be managed with frequent hair washing, either with regular shampoo or any of the over-the-counter preparations available for this purpose.

Occasionally dandruff progresses to a more severe form of dermatitis, with redness and scaling around the ears and eyebrows. The skin creases around the nose and elsewhere may become involved (armpits, groin, anal area), wherever skin folds are located. Especially among obese persons the condition has a tendency to become more severe. In such instances, topical steroids in lotion, cream, or gel form may be helpful. If these lesions become secondarily infected, topical antibiotics or antifungal agents may be necessary, preferably taken under the direction of a physician.

8

The Later Years

Over the past century the average length of human life in the United States has increased greatly; for men it is now 73 years. The reasons are obvious: improvements in health care, nutrition, housing, sanitation, and expanded social service programs.

But age we must, and some do it better than others. True, our genes often program us for baldness or early wrinkles, but we can make the difference when it comes to growing older by our life-styles and health habits.

A Sensible Diet

For years, nutritionists in government and academia have been recommending certain prudent dietary practices for the maintenance of good health. As a result, the needs for limitation of total fat intake, an increase in the proportion of polyunsaturates and monosaturates consumed, and for increased fiber in the diet are well recognized today.

Are vitamins and other dietary supplements recommended

in addition to a normal sensible diet? Most nutritional experts point out that if one adheres to an adequate diet, such supplements are unnecessary. Certainly dietary supplements are popular; surveys indicate that over half of older Americans, especially in retirement homes, routinely dose themselves with vitamins and/or minerals. Given the availability and low cost of most vitamins, there are probably no major objections to taking low dosages of some vitamins. One should avoid the use of **megavitamins** however; extra-large doses of certain vitamin and other nutritional supplements have been shown to be associated with serious and even fatal complications.

Calcium has been recommended for women because of the risk of osteopororis (a weakening of the bones) with advancing age. No similar argument can be made for men—ingestion of calcium in those with adequate stores of this mineral may precipitate kidney stones as well as cause other complications.

As we age, our diets may become deficient in iron. This deficiency might result in anemia and thus justify the routine taking of iron supplements in the diet. The risk of iron-deficiency anemia is greater in older women than in men because of the chronic blood loss from menses during a woman's reproductive life. An iron-deficiency anemia in a man should always raise suspicions of bleeding, possibly from an unsuspected malignancy, ulcer, or other medical condition requiring medical investigation.

Deficiencies of zinc, chromium, and selenium—so-called trace elements because of the small amounts in which they are found within the body—have been linked to certain diseases, but no routine dietary supplements of these minerals have been justified with the present state of our knowledge.

Exercise

Regular exercise can maintain muscle tone, keep weight down, and provide an overall improvement in one's sense of well-being. To the extent that it is not ill-advised on the basis of some underlying disease, some daily exercise is always beneficial. What any man over 40, or perhaps even over 35, should *not* do is suddenly embark on a strenuous exercise program without first consulting a physician about possible risks he may be assuming in starting such a program.

For older men, lesser degrees of exercise will probably suffice: tennis doubles instead of singles; brisk walking instead of jogging or running; swimming instead of arduous workouts with weights.

However, whether because of heredity, bad habits, or just bad luck, all of us eventually will show the effects of our advancing years. Some men unfortunately may be subject to the more serious diseases that normally occur only in the later years—heart disease, arthritis, and eye and hearing complications.

What to Expect

As we grow older, our various body systems begin to show the effects of prolonged wear and tear. These disorders constitute the so-called degenerative diseases of old age, perhaps indicated most clearly in diseases of the joints (arthritis) and in the heart and brain, where the blood vessels may begin to show signs of blockage owing to the accumulated damage of a lifetime of circulating fats within the bloodstream. For those who do not succumb to vascular disease in old age, cancer begins to loom as a more prominent threat.

Not all the differences observed between the young and old are pathological, however. Many are at least in part the result of normal aging. Perhaps the most ambitious study of normal aging has been the one carried out since 1958 at the Gerontology Research Center in Baltimore, now part of the National Institute on Aging. The Baltimore Longitudinal Study of Aging has involved approximately 1,000 men and women, ranging in age from 20 to 96 years. These subjects report periodically from all parts of the country for tests on their physical condition and functioning. Some of the results of such long-term studies of normal aging, as derived from the Baltimore group and elsewhere, are shown in the table below.

Some Effects of Normal Aging in Men

Organ or Function	Finding
Body structure	Loss of height (minor), increase in chest circumference, increase in total body weight (to late 50s), decrease in lean weight (60s and 70s)
Metabolic rate	Decrease
Red blood cells	No change to 65, slight fall thereafter
Cartilage	Loss of elasticity, and deposits of calcium
Muscle mass	Thirty-percent loss by eighth decade
Muscle strength	Decrease after 35
Cardiovascular	Decrease in heart rate, valve rigidity, and calcification, increased stiffness of heart muscle and blood vessels
Respiratory	Diminished function
Kidneys	Decrease in mass, blood flow, and filtration rate after 40
Gastrointestinal	Increase in stomach acid, delay in stomach emptying and intestinal motility
Endocrine	Decrease in glucose tolerance

Illness in Older Men

When geriatric specialists first began to take a close look at our aging male population, it became apparent that significant illness in the elderly was being grossly unreported and unrecognized. Besides the many physical, social, and economic reasons for this situation, many common illnesses tend to be attributed solely to aging, and so nothing is done. In other instances the elderly, especially those with limited resources, recognize that they are ill, but do not wish to add the cost of medical care to an already overburdened budget. Detecting illnesses may be further hampered by the isolation of the elderly, by language barriers, and, in some instances, by preexisting or concomitant mental deterioration that may cause confusion and delay in the reporting of symptoms to family, friends, and physicians. Additionally, the diagnosis of illness among the elderly requires knowledge and skills different from those employed for younger people with the same conditions.

One of the atypical aspects of disease in the elderly involves the effects of infection. One of the first things younger adults do when an infection is suspected is to pull out a thermometer and take their temperature, knowing that fever is often an early symptom. In the elderly, on the other hand, severe, even life-threatening infections may be present without the detection of any temperature elevation, at least not early in the course of the disease.

It also appears that the elderly tolerate pain better. To what degree this is due to a diminished perception of pain, an increased acceptance of it as part of the natural process of aging, or both, varies from person to person. The end result is that pain-producing conditions that may bring a younger patient to the doctor posthaste may be ignored for dangerously long periods by older people.

Another aspect of illness among the elderly is that it is often multiple. For example, the elderly patient with pneumonia may often have diabetes, heart disease, and other health problems complicating the picture and making diagnosis of a new illness more complex and difficult.

Medication

For several reasons, overmedication and undermedication are both special problems among the elderly. Because they often have multiple ailments, the elderly are often subjected to polypharmacy; that is, they are much more likely to be taking several drugs for several conditions. One study of hospitalized Medicare patients showed, for example, that some patients were receiving between three and ten different medications. This all leads to greatly increased opportunities for mishaps, from selecting the inappropriate drugs and dosages to confused compliance by the patient, and unanticipated drug interactions.

Second, the overall incidence of adverse drug reactions in

older persons has been shown to be two to three times that found in young adults, even when the drug is prescribed and administered properly. Most drugs are altered in some way during passage through the liver, and the livers of the elderly may handle drugs differently from those of younger individuals. As well, increased fat deposits among the elderly may alter release patterns, blood levels, and effects of medications administered. Excretion of drugs by the kidneys may also be impaired. The nutritional status of patients is important in the proper handling of medications by the body, and older patients are often subject to poor nutritional states.

Compliance can also be a special problem. Some older patients stop taking their medication when they feel better, thus precipitating multiple acute attacks in chronic conditions that require long-term therapy. Lack of funds may lead to failure to renew prescriptions. Problems with hearing, vision, and mental alertness may create confusion. For the elderly poor who attend public clinics, there is the additional problem that they may see a different doctor each time, with no chance for the doctor to get to know the patient well enough to get past some of these problems of communication. And of course, using many doctors who are trying to manage the same illnesses can lead to conflicting approaches. Often this will only help to fill up a patient's medicine cabinet with medications that should not be taken together but often are.

Those responsible for medicating the elderly—doctors, families, and the patients themselves—must keep these complicating factors in mind.

Several things can be done to avoid risks and alert health-care personnel to an older person's situation:

1. Anyone hiring a caretaker for an elderly person should make sure he or she clearly understands the situation. It's best to put any verbal instructions in writing so there is no room for misunderstanding. This is especially important regarding required dosages and timing of medications.

2. Elderly patients often do not like to follow the doctor's orders, especially if this means changing their life-style or routine. It is important that the caregiver, whether a member of the family or someone hired from outside, is firm with the

patient and is accountable to the physician regarding his or her instructions.

3. Families need to plan ahead and get backup assistance if a hired caregiver doesn't show up or can't come for some reason. They should not take it for granted that family members, neighbors, or friends will automatically step in and help.

4. Family members should check up regularly on elderly parents or relatives who live alone, to make sure they are well, that no new symptoms have occurred, that they are taking their medicine on a scheduled basis, and that they are in touch with a physician at all times. Telephone calls should be supplemented with frequent home visits, if at all possible.

CARDIOVASCULAR DISEASE

Cholesterol levels tend to rise with advancing years, and men over 60 have the highest prevalence of elevated blood cholesterol. The increased risks attending such elevations in terms of developing coronary heart disease are the same as for younger men. Therefore the same attention to diet and the possible use of lipid-lowering agents should be employed for those 60 and beyond as among middle-aged men.

Hypertension

With advancing age, elastic tissue is replaced by fibrous tissue, and the arterial walls become stiff. With each pumping of blood from the heart, the arterial walls are less flexible, and the maximum pressure reached is higher. Our grandparents and their doctors were well aware of this phenomenon; in past years it was assumed that the normal systolic blood pressure should be calculated as 100 plus a person's age.

As a result, isolated systolic blood pressure elevation is common among the elderly and is related even more than diastolic hypertension to coronary problems. This condition should be treated, but two factors complicate the decision for both the older patient and his doctor.

The first is that drug treatment of systolic hypertension in the elderly is often difficult. With aging arteries, as stated before, there is lack of flexibility, and the **baroreceptors** (structures located within the arterial system to modulate any changes in blood pressure) may also become defective. Both factors, following the administration of blood-pressure-lowering drugs, can lead to weakness, dizziness, and fainting.

The second consideration in the treatment of systolic hypertension in the older person is the lack of definitive long-term beneficial effects such as have been clearly demonstrated with the treatment of diastolic hypertension among younger groups. Because of such concerns, those treating systolic hypertension in the elderly do so conservatively. Dietary means to lower pressure, such as weight loss and salt restriction, should be tried before drug therapy is initiated.

Aortic Stenosis

Narrowing of the valve at the juncture of the left ventricle and aorta is a common problem among the elderly. It may result from preexisting rheumatic heart disease involving the valve, even though critical narrowing shows up only late in life. It may be related to a congenital malformation of the aortic valve or to an alteration caused by the normal aging process.

With advancing years there is a tendency for the aortic valve surface to become somewhat roughened, accompanied by minor irregularities of valve shape. Often this is signaled by the appearance of a new heart murmur that in no way reflects any difficulties the valve has in opening and closing. In some instances, however, excessive amounts of calcium salts begin to deposit on the valve cusps, interfering with the valve's ability to open fully as the left ventricle contracts with each heart cycle. This process is accompanied by a murmur in the same area of the chest as that occurring with the previously described totally benign condition. How does the doctor differentiate between the two? Both conditions may be unaccompanied by cardiac symptoms. Some physical findings or the resting electrocardiogram may offer assistance, but these are often incapable of making a clear differentiation.

In the past, many older men who really had nothing amiss were obliged to undergo cardiac catheterization to prove it. Now, fortunately, echocardiography has filled an important need. The character of the aortic valve can be determined, and an accurate estimate can be made of any pressure gradient across the valve between the left ventricle and aorta. This provides valuable information on the severity of the obstruction.

Someone can have severe aortic stenosis without any symptoms. When symptoms do occur they usually are of three types. There may be chest pain (typical angina) resulting from the inability of normal coronary flow to meet the demands of the thickened heart muscle wall that has developed in response to the obstruction. There may be fainting spells resulting from periodic inability of the cardiac output to meet the oxygen demands of the brain. Congestive heart failure may result when the overstressed left ventricle simply gives out. In addition to these, sudden unexpected death is always a threat in severe aortic stenosis.

The only satisfactory treatment of aortic stenosis is surgical relief of the obstruction. This is usually accomplished by replacing the diseased valve with some sort of artificial mechanical valve with one or two tilting discs. An alternative approach is the use of a **bioprosthetic valve** constructed from the specially prepared valves of mammals such as pigs. Sculpturing of the valve without replacement is another option, but may result in significant leakage, so it is not in general use. **Balloon valvuloplasty,** the insertion of a catheter with a balloon mounted on it that is blown up to increase the size of the valve opening, is another option in the critically ill patient who may not be able to withstand major heart surgery.

In the elderly patient, obstructive coronary disease frequently coexists with aortic stenosis, and cardiac catheterization is wise before undertaking the valve surgery. If surgery is elected, bypass surgery can be performed at the same time. Following surgery, long-term anticoagulation medication to prevent clots from forming on the artificial valve is advisable.

Fainting (Syncope)

The sudden loss of consciousness in anyone can be alarming. Among the elderly it is not uncommon, and when it occurs, the search for a cause focuses on the brain and cardiovascular system. In the latter area, aortic stenosis must be considered. Fainting can also result from irregularities in the heartbeat or can be the initial symptom in acute myocardial infarction, which most people call a heart attack.

Another cause of fainting, common in the elderly, is **orthostatic hypotension,** a sudden marked drop in blood pressure. This occurs when you stand or sit upright abruptly and a transient decrease in blood flow to the brain results in a loss of consciousness. Your doctor can easily test for this in the office by measuring blood pressures when you are lying down and standing. Effective treatment includes the use of blocks to elevate the head of the bed, and the more gradual assumption of the standing position. Elastic stockings, extending to the thighs, may occasionally be prescribed. When similar methods fail, the oral form of one of the cortisone family of drugs may be effective. Orthostatic hypotension often represents a side effect of certain medications that then should be reduced or discontinued.

Postmicturition syncope may occur in elderly men. As they stand before the urinal, bearing down to pass urine, their efforts may reduce the return of venous blood to the heart and result in fainting. **Carotid sinus syncope** is the result of excessively sensitive receptors in either of the carotid arteries, which, when stimulated by some external pressure, result in a loss of consciousness.

With increasing age, the conduction system of the heart—its "electrical wiring"—may become diseased. The resulting heart block may cause fainting or even convulsions when heart rates drop below 40 or 45. This is easily diagnosed by electrocardiography, and treated effectively with a permanently implanted pacemaker.

More recently it has been found that among the aging population the primary pacemaker of the heart, the **sinus node,** may go awry, resulting in the **sick sinus syndrome.** Here, very slow heart rates, very fast heart rates, or fast heart rates followed by periods of no activity result in symptoms of erratic blood flow to the brain. Electrophysiological testing can usually pinpoint the cause; again, a permanent cardiac pacemaker usually solves the problem.

Aneurysms

These are abnormal "outpockets" or pouches in the cardio-vascular system caused by a weakened spot in the wall of the heart or artery. In the heart they may be related to a previous heart attack (ventricular aneurysms). More commonly, aneurysmal swellings occur in the main arterial vessel arising from the heart, the aorta. Within the aorta the most common location is in the abdominal portion. They are not uncommon accompaniments to old age. The danger is that they will eventually rupture, with catastrophic consequences. When the aortic aneurysm is accompanied by symptoms, usually pain in the abdomen, flanks, or lower back region, the need for action is clear. It is the asymptomatic abdominal aneurysm—discovered incidentally on routine physical examination or detected by abdominal X rays performed for totally unrelated reasons—that frequently presents difficult choices to the physician.

Measurement of the size of the aneurysm, performed by ultrasound or X-ray techniques, has been the most useful way of evaluating the need for surgery. Those aneurysms having a diameter of five centimeters or more, even when asymptomatic, have a significant likelihood of rupturing. Since surgery performed after a rupture has a much higher mortality, the decision is usually made to operate electively in such patients, replacing the diseased portion of the aorta with a Dacron graft. For smaller aneurysms, the Mayo Clinic group, which has much experience in this field, advises a repeat study three to six months after initial detection, followed by semiannual to annual evaluations.

Stroke

The brain is vitally dependent upon a rich and constant supply of blood. It has been estimated that any deprivation of oxygenated blood to a portion of the brain that exceeds four minutes can result in irreversible damage to nerve cells. A stroke represents the neurological deficit that results from any sudden interruption of blood flow to the brain. Most often it results in **hemiparesis,** a paralysis of one side of the body, reflecting an insult to the opposite side of the brain, since the motor fibers cross within the brain before finally being distributed to the appropriate muscle bundles within the body. Strokes continue to represent a major health problem, about half a million a year occurring within the United States.

There are three major causes of stroke: bleeding within the brain, **thrombosis** (blood clotting) within an artery that delivers blood within the brain, and obstruction of one of these same arteries by a clot that has formed elsewhere—usually the heart—and that has broken off and traveled to a vital artery within the brain. This last condition is called a **cerebral embolism.**

Bleeding can occur at any age with severe uncontrolled hypertension, resulting in accumulating blood pressing upon and destroying the brain tissue. Vascular malformations within the brain may be present from birth but remain totally unsuspected until they cause a brain hemorrhage. Such catastrophes, which can be fatal, often occur in early to middle life, with no previous warning symptoms.

Among the elderly it is blood clotting or cerebral thrombosis that accounts for the majority of strokes, 80 percent of them after the age of 75. The third type of vascular insult to the brain, cerebral embolism, has long been recognized as a complication of some forms of rheumatic heart disease in which a combination of low flow and possibly inflammation lead to the formation of clots within the left atrium (see Figure 2.1, page 38). This is especially true when a particular irregularity of the heartbeat called **atrial fibrillation** occurs. In many instances the clots will break off and travel through the left ventricle, out the aorta, and into the vessels of the brain. For years, patients falling into this high-risk category have been given medications to prevent clot formation or have undergone surgery, or both.

Given the relative rarity of rheumatic heart disease today in the United States, it was felt until recently that older people were not at risk of cerebral embolism. Careful long-term studies in several centers throughout the world, however, have now indicated rather strongly that the elderly with atrial fibrillation are also at a high risk for **thrombo-embolism** (clots occurring in the heart). Despite several problems with long-term anticoagulation therapy—the need for repeated testing for control, the expense of the medications used, and the small but definite risk of causing accidental bleeding in the brain—more and more doctors are advising such therapy in these cases.

Selection of the proper drug remains somewhat controversial. It would be fortunate if simple aspirin alone did the job, but some studies indicate that full anticoagulation with **warfarin** (Coumadin) may be necessary.

What happens after a stroke? First there must be some effort to determine the cause of the stroke and take measures to prevent a recurrence if possible. Equally important is the need for early and intensive rehabilitative therapy. Motion exercises will prevent contractures, the freezing up of joints due to neurological damage affecting associated muscle groups. Use of braces, canes, and walkers is essential. Special speech, physical, and occupational therapies also make important contributions in striking back at stroke. With such efforts, many stroke victims can regain an appreciable return of function, although complete recovery is rare.

Transient Ischemic Attacks (TIAs)

Because of the devastating impact of stroke upon any individual, any warning sign of an impending event is, in a certain sense, welcome. "Little strokes" or TIAs fall into this category. These are defined as transient neurological deficits that appear and then disappear within a 24-hour period, although most last only 15 minutes or less. They can be manifested as passing numbness or weakness of an extremity, usually the hand. There may be transient slurring of speech, inappropriate speech, or loss of eyesight.

Many of these episodes are not related to disease within the brain itself but rather in the carotid arteries, the major vessels running through the neck delivering blood to the brain. A popular theory holds that when the walls of these arteries become roughened with atherosclerotic plaques there is an accumulation of tiny collections of blood platelets or fibrin, a blood protein. These aggregates break off periodically and travel to small vessels of the brain where they shut down the blood supply downstream and cause the symptoms typical of TIAs.

In order to determine how best to treat this disorder, the

physician may employ a number of diagnostic tests. Initially, noninvasive testing helps to mark the location and suggest the severity of obstructions. The standard diagnosis, however, involves the invasive procedure of angiography, in which a catheter is introduced into an artery, usually in the groin, and passed retrogradely so that the tip is located near the points at which the major vessels to the head, including the carotids, branch off. Radiopaque material is then injected through the catheter to outline the vessels.

Carotid angiography, as it is called, unfortunately is not a completely benign procedure. Serious complications occur in approximately 1 to 2 percent of studies, and include stroke and even death. There can be bleeding and damage to the arteries—troublesome complications of a procedure that is, after all, diagnostic and not therapeutic. Because of such considerations, the technique of **digital subtraction angiography** (DIVA) was developed as a possible substitute for conventional angiography. Here the contrast media is injected in a peripheral vein rather than an artery, with repeated films of the carotid vessels taken as they fill with the outlining material. Unfortunately the test has proved insufficiently reliable for diagnostic purposes, and unsuspected complications have occurred with it as well. As a result, it is gradually falling out of favor.

Once the location and degree of obstruction is determined, a decision must be made as to whether medical or surgical treatment will best serve the interests of the patient. For minor irregularities in the wall of a carotid artery, aspirin, which reduces the stickiness of platelets, is the accepted treatment. In elderly men, especially, it has been found that the incidence of subsequent stroke can be reduced by about 30 percent by taking aspirin on a regular basis. Untreated, patients with TIAs stand a 10-percent chance of stroke within the first year following an attack, with a 3-to-5-percent incidence in subsequent years.

There are some lesions that may be better treated surgically. Suitability for surgery depends upon the severity of obstruction, the location of the obstruction (can the surgeon get to it easily?), and a confirming match of the location of the obstruction with the areas of the brain and body affected.

The procedure, **carotid endarterectomy,** involves opening up the vessel and clearing it of the obstructing material, occasionally with the insertion of a patch to enlarge the size of the vessel.

In many instances, however, it is not totally clear which might be the preferred therapy, and it is in such instances that a great deal of disagreement may arise among professionals. Complicating the picture is the fact that carotid endarterectomy is not always without complications, and the risk of such complications varies widely depending on who does the procedure and where it is done.

Noises in the neck. With partial obstruction of the carotids, as occurs in TIAs, there are often sounds or **bruits** heard in the neck arteries, raising initial suspicions of disease located in arteries outside the skull (extracranial arteries). However, even minor obstructions that do not really interfere with blood flow, or even a slight roughening of the arterial wall due to plaques that occur with aging, may create turbulent blood flow and create sounds that can be heard by your doctor when he or she listens through a stethoscope placed over the neck vessels.

Carotid bruits in asymptomatic elderly individuals are not rare, occurring in about 5 percent of those 75 and older. They carry with them an increased risk of subsequent stroke, about two and a half times that in those who do not have the condition. In the past there was a tendency, especially in this country, to investigate such patients thoroughly, with the intention of performing endarterectomy in selected cases before a stroke might occur.

Arguing against such management was the finding that about half of these patients who did have strokes had them in relation to disease within the brain and not related to obstructions in the carotid artery. When the risks and expense of invasive diagnosis and surgery were added in, there was a growing feeling that these outweighed any fears of an increased risk of stroke on the basis of carotid disease. The weight of current medical opinion is to abstain from these procedures in the asymptomatic individual with a carotid bruit. Nonetheless, he or she should be observed closely for any signs of difficulty.

As might be gathered from the foregoing discussion, the management of carotid disease constitutes one of the most controversial issues in protecting the health of the elderly. The results of the many prospective studies now being carried on throughout the world are anxiously anticipated by patients and doctors alike.

ARTHRITIC AND ORTHOPEDIC PROBLEMS

Difficulties with degenerative joint disease are particularly prominent among older people. Another condition, one only recently being recognized as a problem for those 60 years of age and older, is **calcium pyrophospate deposition disease** (CPPD). By the age of 72, about 6 percent of the adult population will have these crystals in their joints; an estimated 3 to 20 percent of the geriatric population may develop symptoms as a result of this condition.

Although there is a chronic "smoldering" form of the disease, most often the onset of symptoms is sudden and severe, resembling another condition of the joints, acute gout. **Pseudo-gout** is the term used to describe CPPD when it occurs in this manner. The means of differentiation lies in analysis of the types of crystals in the joint fluid. Over time there may be typical appearances of these crystals on X-ray films to help differentiate CPPD from true gout.

The pain in an acute attack of pseudo-gout is most often in the knee rather than the base of the big toe. When mistaken for true gout, it is sometimes treated with colchicine, but the response is not the same as in gout. Injecting steroids directly into the joint space seems to be the most effective way to control it, along with other general methods of pain relief, including analgesics.

NEUROLOGICAL AND MENTAL CHANGES

What happens to our mental faculties as we age? A popular conception is that we slow down, forget recent events, and tend to remember those deep in the past—the latter almost too well, according to the young. Studies made over the course of several decades are showing that it is not quite as simple as that.

Actually, up to the age of 70, intellectual performance, in the main, remains intact. It is only at that point that our mental processing begins to slow down. To a great extent this is compensated by the excellent judgment that a wealth of previous experience has supplied the older individual, especially in arriving at important life-style decisions.

Interestingly enough, constant exercising of the mind throughout one's life seems to have the same kind of conditioning effect on the brain that physical exercise has on the muscles of the body. Creative and intellectual people seem to pass 70 without experiencing any diminution of the vigor of their thought processes. About a quarter of the population approaching 80 will show no signs of memory loss or inability to think clearly.

With all the advances in medicine, public health, sanitation, nutrition, and improvement in working conditions over the past decades, it is highly likely that the 70-year-old man in the 1990s is better equipped biologically to face the succeeding years than was his counterpart in the 1920s. Now we know, however, that much of the mental disability seen in the elderly is not simply an aspect of growing old, but rather caused by illness or a specific form of dementia known as Alzheimer's disease.

Alzheimer's Disease

Dementia is a general term for mental deterioration, which can include loss of memory, mental flexibility, language, and other intellectual faculties, including normal emotional and behavioral responses. Alzheimer's disease (AD) is a form of senile dementia that affects about 4 million Americans a year, at a cost to the economy of between $24 billion and $48 billion annually. The prevalence of AD increases with advancing age. A recent study conducted in Boston showed a rise in prevalence from 3 percent of the population between 65 and 74 to 19 percent of people aged 75 to 84, up to 47 percent in those over 85. With an increasingly aging population, the problem can only become worse in the future.

Alzheimer's disease was first described by Dr. Alois Alzheimer in 1907, when he examined the brain of a woman who inexplicably demonstrated rapid and progressive mental deterioration over a period of nearly five years prior to her death. He found, upon microscopic examination, a number of abnormal structures (senile plaques) within the brain, combined with a prominent display of twisted nerve elements (neurofibrillary tangles). The disease also caused a 20-to-40-percent loss of nerve cells, reflected in atrophy or shrinkage of the brain.

There is a genetically related form of AD, with first-degree relatives (children, brothers, and sisters) five times more likely to develop it than others in the general population. This accounts for only about 10 percent of those affected, however. For the overwhelming majority at risk, the selection is random and the cause unknown. There has been no infectious agent found responsible, and no specific environmental factor identified, although aluminum toxicity was suspected at one time.

The onset of Alzheimer's disease is insidious, almost imperceptible. A previously normal individual, usually in his or her late fifties or early sixties, begins to experience slight losses of memory. At first this is unnoticed or denied until its further progression results in an unmistakable recognition of the individual's mental deterioration. Employment becomes impossible, and those affected become increasingly dependent upon family and friends for any semblance of normal daily functioning. Inability to walk or eat properly occurs, and urinary and bowel incontinence are also common at later stages. Although the course of AD can be quite variable, death, usually from a kidney or lung infection, usually occurs between five and 10 years after the onset of the disease.

Although the pathological features of AD are rather typical, there is no specific blood test that can be performed during one's life that will make the diagnosis. The mental deterioration seen in AD could be an indication of other mental disorders, some of which are amenable to specific therapy. For this reason, CT scanning of the brain has proved very helpful in distinguishing AD from some of these other conditions.

A further refinement in diagnosis may be provided by **positron emission tomography** (PET). While the information obtained from CT scans is purely anatomical, PET provides physicians with information about the metabolic and biochemical functioning of the brain. Metabolically active substances such as glucose are tagged radioactively and then injected intravenously into the patient. Other radioactive tags can indicate patterns of blood flow in the brain substance. Following these injections, scanning can reveal abnormalities of the brain.

Is there any effective medical therapy for AD? In the early 1980s, attempts were made to enhance nerve transmission with certain drugs then available, but these have not proved effective. Later the drug **hydergine** was felt to be a "metabolic enhancer" that improved the function of nerve cells and transmission of nervous activity. Currently the only drug for AD approved by the Food and Drug Administration, and one of the most commonly prescribed drugs throughout the world, hydergine too may prove a failure in AD. A recent rigorous collaborative study from the University of Colorado and the Jefferson Medical College, in Philadelphia, has failed to show any positive effect of hydergine on AD, even with an improved formulation of the drug.

Investigators continue to work on **beta amyloid,** a component of the senile plaques found in the brains of deceased victims of AD. The potential uses of **nerve growth factor,** a naturally occurring protein necessary for nerve growth, are also being explored. The genetics of AD are being examined to determine its exact cause or causes, and perhaps provide clues to future therapy. A deficiency of **corticotropin-releasing hormone,** important for nerve transmission, has been found in AD patients. Perhaps this will provide an avenue for future therapy.

For the present, a therapy to truly reverse the disease remains strictly theoretical and only within the confines of the research laboratory. Most drugs currently prescribed are mainly for the purpose of reducing some of the disruptive and disabling symptoms of the disease.

Perhaps more rewarding are the attempts being made to maintain the socialization of AD victims by providing assistance in their daily activities. "Reminiscence" group therapy seems to help in maintaining a patient's orientation, and day-care centers are proving an essential component to long-term management of this progressive disease. Self-help groups have been established nationwide to help those newly introduced to the problems of caring for the AD patient, and they are proving invaluable.

Parkinsonism

In 1817 Sir James Parkinson described a kind of "shaking palsy" among his older patients. Today it is estimated that this disease, Parkinsonism, affects 1 percent of the population over the age of 50. This translates into about one million Americans. Although there are several causes of the disorder, the most common is a degeneration of certain nerves within the brain, which results in a decrease in **dopamine,** a brain substance.

The effects of this deficiency on the individual are tremor, rigidity, and difficulty in walking. Tremor in the hands is one of the most recognizable features of the disease. Perhaps even more common is the characteristic rigidity, a lack of normal movement in the arm, and a stiffness in the face that gives it a masklike appearance. **Bradykinesia,** literally "slow motion," is the term that describes the difficulty with which the patient initiates and carries out everyday movements such as walking, writing, and all those hand movements involved in a wide variety of daily functions. A typical shuffling gait, characterized by a rigid, forward-bent posture and abrupt, unsteady starts and stops, is the final prominent, easily recognizable feature of Parkinsonism.

The course of the disease's progression is variable, but it is frequently prolonged and results in long-term disability for those affected. Recently a number of younger patients in their thirties and forties have started appearing with Parkinsonism. This has suggested to some investigators that an environmental factor may be at work.

Treatment for this incurable condition was highly unsatisfactory until the introduction of the wonder drug of the late 1960s, **levodopa** (Sinemet, Larodopa), which was found to alleviate the symptoms of the disease, at least for a time. Since then, other, similar drugs called **dopamine agonists** have been introduced, but none of these actually halts progression of the disease.

The newest development in the medical treatment of Parkinsonism is the drug **Deprenyl.** The hope once was that the new medication might halt the progression of the disease and thereby prolong life. Although Deprenyl is effective and a first-line drug for Parkinsonism, it has not lived up to these high expectations. Since the disease is progressive, an end point will probably be reached with Deprenyl as with most medical therapy, when no further improvement can be expected. It is this consideration that led first Swedish researchers and then others to seek the solution with transplantation surgery.

Part of the adrenal gland contains cells that produce dopamine. It was felt that if part of this gland could be transplanted to the Parkinsonism patient's brain, the deficiency of dopamine in the central nervous system could be reversed. After much promising animal experimentation, Swedish surgeons attempted the procedure in patients, but without success. Then, in 1987, Mexican surgeons, using a somewhat different adrenal transplant technique, reported remarkable results with this surgery in a number of patients with Parkinsonism. Their before-and-after videotapes, widely shown in medical circles throughout the world, raised new hopes for this surgical approach in Parkinsonism. Trials were begun in 15 different surgical centers in the United States, but thus far they have not been able to reproduce the results of the Mexicans, and the operation is falling out of favor.

The most recent chapter in the surgical treatment of Parkinsonism again involves the Swedes, who have reported one case of marked improvement in a man receiving a transplant of nervous tissue obtained from aborted fetuses. It is too early to determine what this will portend for the future management of this increasingly problematic disease.

Depression

Within the general population, major depression is actually less of a problem in the 65-and-older group than among younger individuals. One exception to this is the elderly in nursing homes and other long-term care facilities, where between 10 and 20 percent of the elderly patients experience major depressions.

It is older patients, moreover, in whom a major depression can lead to an increased possibility of suicide. In fact, the suicide rate for elderly white men is higher than for any other segment of society. Fortunately, in the absence of other mental disease, depression can usually be managed successfully. Removal of potentially offending medications, rearrangement of environmental conditions, and psychiatric assistance, usually short-term, can combine to resolve most depression problems in this group.

OTHER SYSTEMIC CHANGES

As we age, certain changes may occur in vital body systems that we once took for granted. Many of these dysfunctions, however, are receiving increased attention as the population ages; adequate treatment now exists to relieve symptoms or prevent further damage or disability related to these conditions.

Urinary Functions

Incontinence. At least 10 million Americans are affected with urinary incontinence, including 15 to 30 percent of the elderly living independently, and at least half of those in nursing homes. This problem can no longer be ignored.

In the past no medical basis could be found for most cases of incontinence—a necessary first step in attempting effective treatment. The common practice of supplying adult diapers for those in and out of nursing homes, and of sticking catheters into the bladders of those confined, is neither a sane nor humane approach to the problem. At last those concerned with the delivery of optimum health care are beginning to rectify this deplorable situation.

Normal urinary continence in men depends upon a number of factors. These include a compliant bladder; properly functioning nerves and muscles within the bladder and around the urethra that help in the normal storage of urine; and, finally, normal mental function to control the process of urination.

Several specific patterns of urinary incontinence have been recognized; in about one-third of those affected, a combination of these may exist. **Stress incontinence** occurs when pressure within the abdominal cavity exceeds that within the bladder, and inadequate sphincter control at the neck of the bladder allows for escape of urine. This commonly occurs with coughing and with activities such as bearing down to lift heavy objects off the floor. **Urge incontinence** occurs when the need to urinate is sensed, but the individual cannot get to the toilet in time and an involuntary passage of urine occurs. Post-stroke patients may experience this, as well as those with other neurological diseases. In others with urge incontinence, however, no specific neurological defect can be pinpointed.

Overflow incontinence occurs when the bladder cannot empty normally and becomes overdistended, with urine dribbling out past a certain maximal capacity. Such is the case in benign prostatic hypertrophy, although strictures of the urethra and other structural abnormalities can result in this pattern. **Functional incontinence** occurs when there is no essential defect in the urinary system, but external factors, such as being bedridden, interfere with getting to the toilet, resulting in "accidents."

Individuals suffering from urinary incontinence should undergo thorough physical examination to determine accurately the character of their complaint. A urologist should be consulted for the most precise diagnosis and treatment. A number of treatment programs, noninvasive as well as invasive, are currently available. For example, certain bladder relaxants can help in the control of urgency incontinence. Drugs that strengthen bladder outlet function may also help. Surgery may be indicated for obstructions such as those related to benign prostatic hypertrophy.

When intellectual function is impaired, such as occurs in Alzheimer's disease, urinary incontinence may simply be a reflection of this impairment. In such cases, little is to be expected from therapy aimed at the incontinence itself. On the other hand, many elderly men are perfectly capable, intellectually, of cooperating to get this disturbing condition under control.

Behavior modification is one technique that has demonstrated success in such instances. Special exercises have been widely used in women to strengthen pelvic muscles and control stress incontinence, and now there is evidence to support the efficacy of such exercises in men as well. Biofeedback techniques that utilize visual or auditory instrumentation to tell patients how well they are controlling bladder function can be very useful. With stress incontinence and/or urge incontinence, complete recovery has been reported in 20 to 25 percent of patients, with another one-third demonstrating significant improvement of their symptoms.

The growing importance of this problem has been recognized by the establishment of the International Continence Society for the study of this disorder. Meanwhile, lay organizations such as HIP (Help for Incontinent People) and the Simon Foundation address the problem on the community level.

Constipation

Complaints about constipation increase with aging. There are several causes for this: diets that are low in fiber; sedentary habits; medications that interfere with normal bowel function; and a number of diseases common among the elderly that interfere with the normal nerve and muscle function associated with defecation. The most important factor regulating proper formation of stool is dietary: Adequate fiber and fluid in the diet are essential. Many medications play a role in causing constipation that may progress to fecal impaction. Although constipation may be a sign of mental depression, some of the drugs used to treat depression (tricyclic antidepressants, phenothiazines) can themselves cause the problem. Some drugs used to treat hypertension also may cause constipation. Diuretics, prescribed because they remove excess salt and water, may also result in dehydration and poor stool formation.

Prevention of constipation is an important component of normal health care, especially in the elderly, but fixation upon the bowels is not the answer. Overconcern about daily regularity of bowel movements serves no useful purpose. A bowel movement every day is not a requirement of normal health; three or four bowel movements a week are perfectly adequate for almost everyone.

A sensible approach to normal health practice regarding bowel function should, first of all, include the adequate intake of fiber and fluid. Exercise, or at least efforts to maintain close-to-normal physical activity, should be pursued. Removal or reduction of medications that precipitate constipation is mandatory.

Changes in Sexual Function

Although there is a normal decline in sexual activity as men grow older, a great deal of variability exists in this area of our lives. Men who were sexually active in their earlier years will be more likely to maintain a reasonable amount of sexual activity at 60 and beyond, although the number and strength of erections may diminish, and the period between erections becomes prolonged.

Marriage seems to be conducive to the prolongation of sexual vigor in men. In a 1990 survey conducted in Michigan among the elderly, 74 percent of married men were continuing an active sexual life, compared with only 31 percent of men who were unmarried. Interestingly, when various other social and behavioral factors were analyzed, the consumption of one or more cups of coffee a day was associated with increased sexual activity for both sexes. The chemical or physiological basis for this seeming aphrodisiac effect of a beverage that has frequently been medically maligned (often unjustly) is unexplained.

Such findings in married men, especially those who are coffee drinkers, do not obscure the fact that impotence can be a problem for the aging man. In the Baltimore Longitudinal Study of Aging, it has been found that an overall impotence rate of 8 percent among younger men jumps to 25 percent at the age of 65, 55 percent at 75, and 75 percent for those 80 and older. In the vast majority of instances, impotence in the older man is the result of some physical problem rather than a psychological one. For this reason an older man who suddenly begins to experience problems with potency should not hesitate to broach the subject to his physician to detemine what possible physical impediment might exist, and what might be done about it.

It should be emphasized that age should not automatically be equated with impotence. Remember that nearly half the men at 75 in the Baltimore study were still sexually active; your chances of falling into this category as that age approaches are not bad at all.

CHANGES IN THE SENSES

Vision

The need for corrective glasses as we age goes almost without saying. More severe and potentially damaging effects on eyesight, especially among the elderly, are related to three major conditions: cataracts, glaucoma, and macular degeneration.

Cataracts. These are growing opacities of the lens of the eye. They are present to some extent in more than 95 percent of those over 65. When minor, they may not noticeably interfere with vision. When they become severe, however, they must be removed surgically. In the past, thick glasses were required postoperatively to replace the function of the lens that was removed. Today, eye surgeons can substitute implantable artificial lenses instead of having to prescribe unsightly cataract spectacles.

Glaucoma. In this condition, a buildup of fluid within the eyeball results in an elevated pressure, which damages the optic nerve at the back of the eye, resulting in eventual blindness. There are two kinds of glaucoma. The acute form, which accounts for only 5 to 10 percent of the total, is accompanied by a rapid development of eye pain and hazy vision that calls immediate attention to the condition, a true medical emergency. Medications may help, but surgery may be necessary.

Most commonly, glaucoma occurs in a chronic form, insidious in its onset and detected only through periodic examinations by ophthalmologists or optometrists sensitive to the possibility of this condition, especially among older patients. Whether initially discovered by an ophthalmologist or an optometrist, once discovered, chronic glaucoma is treated only by an ophthalmologist. It is detected in its early stages by a rising pressure within the eyeball as measured by a **tonometer,** a pressure-measuring instrument placed on the surface of the eye following the instillation of a local anesthetic. With the assistance of an **ophthalmoscope**, the examiner can inspect the back of the eye to ascertain the appearance of the optic disk (the endings of the optic nerve in the eye). Testing for alterations in visual fields—how wide the range of vision is—is also part of the examination.

When treatment is indicated, it is first medical, in the form of drops that will either facilitate drainage of fluid from the eye chamber or inhibit formation of fluid. Either way, the volume of fluid within the eye is decreased, with a resulting fall in pressure. The need for this treatment should be considered lifelong. In about 10 percent of cases the condition will not be controlled by medication, and a surgical procedure to allow better drainage will have to be performed.

Macular degeneration. The major proportion of irreversible loss of vision among those over 65 results from this condition. The **macula lutea** is that portion of the retina at the back of the eye most sensitive to visual impulses and thus responsible for the maximal sharpness of vision obtainable. In some persons of advancing age, it is believed that a dimishing blood supply to this region results in its deterioration. The result is a loss of sight.

Laser treatment may help to delay or restrict this downhill process. Although patients at the end stage of this condition are considered legally blind, the preservation of other portions of the visual apparatus often allows them to function without too much difficulty.

Hearing

Approximately 25 percent of persons 65 and older complain of hearing problems. Screening of older people with devices to measure their acuity reveals a hearing loss in more than one-third.

Despite the loss in appreciation and quality of life that often accompanies this deficit, it has been found that only 25 percent of those with hearing losses actually receive or use hearing aids. In the elderly with loss of intellectual function (senile dementia), especially, a connection has been made between a loss of mental capacity and the loss of hearing. Restoration of normal or improved hearing has been shown to help ameliorate such conditions in some people.

Complicating the problem is the fact that many doctors do not routinely screen for hearing defects; 80 percent do not, in one survey of primary-care physicians. Thus the burden of perceiving and seeking the evaluation of, and treatment for, hearing loss is likely to fall on the individual himself, or on his family.

The following signs should cause a person or his family to suspect hearing loss:

- the use of excessive volume on the radio or television
- loud speech patterns in conversation
- frequent requests of others to repeat what they said
- leaning forward to hear, or bending the "good ear" in the direction of the speaker

The physician who deals with hearing problems is the **otolaryngologist**. Physical examination and audiological testing under his or her professional guidance will reveal the type and severity of hearing loss.

In general, there are two types of hearing loss: conductive deafness and perceptive or sensoneural deafness. **Conductive deafness** relates to problems with the external or middle ear. They can vary from simple wax buildup to a damaged eardrum as a result of past infections, to fixation or immobility of the tiny bones within the middle ear. **Perceptive deafness** refers to actual damage of the nerve fibers responsible for carrying sound impulses to the brain.

Treatment depends upon the cause. Sometimes simple removal of earwax will suffice. Immobilization of the bones of the middle ear, however, may require microsurgical techniques. For conductive problems unrelieved by other methods, and for perceptive hearing loss, a variety of hearing devices are available that can be tailored to the individual's problem.

Perhaps the most remarkable of these is the **cochlear implant,** in use for only about the last decade. This is used for damage that cannot be compensated by ordinary hearing aids. A tiny receiving device is implanted in the mastoid bone behind the ear. Electrodes connect the implant to the cochlear canal. The setup is completed by an external pickup device some weeks after the initial surgery.

Information about the various types of hearing loss and approved devices for their correction is in a booklet entitled *Hearing Aids*, obtained by writing to Department of Veterans Affairs, Veterans Health Services and Research Administration, Washington, DC 20420. Or call the Better Hearing Institute (800-EAR WELL).

A MIRACLE DRUG?

Given the importance of recognizing the signs of advancing age, is it reasonable to expect a "cure" for it? If there is anything even remotely resembling the elixir of life, it is probably **human growth hormone**. In the past the only source of this substance was actual human tissue, and the small supply of this precious material was used to prevent dwarfism in children with growth hormone deficiency. With the miracle of recombinant DNA technology, growth hormone can now be produced in large amounts, and other potential medical uses for it are being explored.

With advancing age there tends to be a decrease in growth hormone production. This results in a loss of lean tissue, an accumulation of fatty tissue, aging of the skin, and decreasing bone density—all recognizable signs of advancing age. Investigators at the Medical College of Wisconsin have found that after six months of injecting growth hormone under the skin of elderly healthy men, these effects could be reversed or improved.

What are the practical implications of this finding? To begin with, don't go rushing to the drugstore or your doctor's office to demand a supply. Growth hormone is not without its problems. It promotes glucose intolerance and therefore can aggravate or induce diabetes. Symptoms of arthralgia or arthritis may be caused by growth hormone, and it can have adverse effects on the cardiovascular system, causing hypertension and even congestive heart failure.

And it's very expensive. Until the true benefits of growth hormone or any other new "miracle" drug can be delineated, your efforts to "stay young" are better expended in more conventional approaches to the maintenance of good health in your later years.

GROWING OLDER IN THE UNITED STATES

The annual cost of health care in the United States rose from $248 billion in 1980 to $647 billion in 1990, an increase from 9.2 to 11.9 percent of the gross national product over the past decade. With the aging of the population and the relatively great demands this segment makes upon total medical care resources, an increase to about 15 percent of GNP can be expected by the year 2000.

A comparison with Canada and many Western European countries reveals that they are devoting about 6 to 8.5 percent of their gross national product to health care. Since the health of people in these countries is no worse than it is here, and is often better, the question is, To what useful purpose is so much money being expended in the United States?

Certainly these are the kinds of questions that our legislators and health-care officials and planners continue to ask, with good reason. They are also the kind of questions that engage the concern of philosophers and medical ethicists. Finally, they are the concerns that families of the terminally ill (often the elderly) and their doctors must struggle with every day in the most palpable and personal ways.

Another often-asked question concerns the advisability of needlessly prolonging the life of someone at the end of an incurable and often painful illness. Frequently this question focuses on the decision to attempt to revive a patient who has experienced a cardiac arrest. It must be recognized that this is almost always a fruitless endeavor in the terminally ill elderly. A multihospital Boston study, reported in 1989, of more than 500 patients over 70 years of age who underwent cardiopulmonary resuscitation, found that only 19, or 3.8 percent, survived to hospital discharge.

Is it really in the best interests of the patient to prolong his or her final agonies in this way? Are the additional few days in intensive care, with such dismal results and at a cost of many thousands of dollars, really worth the price? What about the drainage on limited hospital resources that this might entail? What about the other patients, with possibly better prognoses, denied access to limited resources as a result of such actions?

Such concerns have led some to call for a rationing of health care, a step that is directed primarily at the elderly infirm. However, as Dr. Norman G. Levinsky has pointed out, the high cost of hospital admissions for the elderly accounts for no more than 3.5 percent of Medicare expenses for this group. If Medicare costs for the elderly are to be substantially reduced, this would have to involve the withholding of *routine* care, a policy that would be hard to justify.

Other decisions about the extent of health care are strictly personal. When the individual is mentally competent, he should make sure his instructions are relayed to his doctor, who is duty-bound, within reason and the limits of the law, to follow them. When the patient is mentally incompetent or unconscious, the burden shifts to the families and the doctors concerned. Now *they* must decide whether or not certain diagnostic or therapeutic measures should be undertaken. Ultimately it may come to the decision of whether a "do not resuscitate" order is to be written in the event of a cardiac arrest. This is an enormous responsibility for all concerned.

How can loved ones decide that nothing more should be done for one of their own? Similarly, the doctor may say, "I am sworn to uphold life and dedicated to maintaining it. How can I participate in the decision to end it?" Furthermore, many physicians, sensitive to the potential threat of malpractice suits, are reluctant to take such steps, even though it is doubtful that any have ever been found guilty of criminal neglect under such circumstances.

To relieve or ease the burden of such decisions, many individuals, while still in a state of mental competency, are beginning to write **living wills.** Simply stated, these wills express an individual's desires as to the conditions under which life support would no longer be wanted, and to whom that decision is to be entrusted. These wills do not have to be complicated legal documents; often a simple signed statement, dated and preferably witnessed, is sufficient.

Although recognized in most states, living wills do have a few drawbacks. They are legally binding only for terminal illness, which may be difficult to define at times, and they do not cover persistent vegetative states such as severe dementia or coma.

Because of these deficiencies, some people have opted for **durable powers of attorney** for their health care. These are more flexible and allow a family member or friend to make decisions for one who at some later date may become mentally incompetent.

A power of attorney must at least be notarized, and may

require legal advice and assistance. If you are interested in taking such a step, you should discuss it carefully with legal counsel as well as with the designated surrogate.

Forms for making out living wills and medical powers of attorney can be obtained from The Society for the Right to Die, 250 West 57th Street, New York, NY 10107.

Anyone who wishes to know whether the state they live in permits the use of living wills should call the social services department of their local hospital. Social workers and other personnel should know the regulations of their particular state regarding this matter.

RETIREMENT

Despite the country's many economic problems, we remain a relatively affluent society in which more people seem to be retiring at an earlier age. In some cases this is involuntary. Physical or mental illness may preclude the continuation of gainful employment. Or a man just past 50 may work in a factory that is suddenly shut down, at which point he finds the job market closed to him. He may own his own home, have close ties to the local community, and decide to retire.

In other instances the decision to retire early may be elective. Perhaps, upon reaching 50, a man has seen his children through college and into the workplace. His pension and savings seem more than adequate for his future needs. Perhaps he has been offered a good price for his business. It might seem a good time to cash in his chips and retire.

There are important caveats to such a decision. With at least another 20 years of living ahead of him, and given the normal inflationary pressures over time, what seems sufficient now might not meet his needs 10 or 20 years hence. His physician might be concerned with other aspects of early retirement.

Many doctors have been confronted in their offices by depressed older men, still basically vigorous in every respect, who have sprouted a variety of physical or emotional complaints stemming from the inactivity and boredom of premature retirement. There are exceptions to the rule, but in general the wisest course is to keep working as long as you enjoy it and as long as you can.

So much has been written about the problems of aging that there is a tendency to overlook the joys and satisfactions of later life. Enjoying our later years will not depend so much on science curing our illnesses after they occur, but on our practicing sensible and healthy habits that can help us to achieve a long, productive, and fulfilling life.

9

How to Choose a Doctor and Work with the Health-Care System

The circumstances giving rise to your search for medical care may vary. Perhaps your old physician has died or retired. For one reason or another you may be dissatisfied with your current doctor and want to find a new one. You may recently have moved to a new location and want to find a local physician to oversee your medical care in the future.

All the above are nonemergency conditions, so you can approach the problem on a systematic basis, taking your time to make the right decision. (In case of an emergency, you should go immediately to the emergency room of the best hospital in your area.)

When choosing a physician for your long-term care, you should take a number of factors into account. Do you prefer a male or female physician? Would you feel more comfortable with an older, established, experienced physician or with a younger doctor, who may be a little more energetic and—perhaps more important—available without a large established practice competing for his or her attention. Are you committed to the idea of the traditional general practitioner who knows something about a lot of things, or are you more comfortable in the hands of a specialist?

With the end of World War II and the explosion of medical knowledge that came along at that time, the Norman Rockwell image of the relaxed family physician faded from the scene. He was replaced by a stream of busy specialists—internist, surgeon, pediatrician, obstetrician-gynecologist. As accumulated knowledge about diseases became even more voluminous and methods to apply it more complex, the subspecialties sprouted forth—cardiologists, heart surgeons, endocrinologists, fertility experts.

What has happened to the patient, with this seemingly irresistible fragmentation of his care? In the minds of many, including some leaders of organized medicine, the patient often became simply a collection of organ systems, each the province of a separate medical expert.

THE PRIMARY-CARE PHYSICIAN

To reverse this trend, the key emphasis in recent years has been on the primary-care physician as opposed to the tertiary-care physician. The primary-care physician is the one you first go to with your symptoms, the one responsible for your general care and long-term medical welfare. The tertiary physician is the specialist to whom the patient may be referred for certain procedures, often surgical in nature. ("Secondary care" has somehow never entered this particular lexicon, perhaps because of that term's other connotations.)

Those who practice internal medicine have long considered themselves the primary-care physicians for adults, as pediatricians have assumed a similar role for children.

THE SPECIALIST

Given the complicated nature of modern medical care, many men cannot accept the premise that any one family physician has the broad range of knowledge and experience necessary to care adequately for every type of illness. A patient, for example, who has had a coronary attack may prefer that a cardiologist be involved in his care. If you have diabetes, you may want the services of an endocrinologist.

Furthermore, a specialist can treat many other types of commonly occurring diseases. Should a patient of a cardiologist or endocrinologist develop pneumonia, bronchitis, or a kidney infection, for example, these specialists are perfectly capable of treating him and, except in rare instances, routinely do so. The downside is that the specialist may tend to ascribe the patient's new complaint to his own area of expertise even when the cause lies elsewhere.

Of course, the importance of having a physician for the whole family may override any deficiencies this physician might have in certain specialized areas. In some of the more isolated areas of the United States, there may be only one physician of any kind within an area of several hundred square miles. In such relatively sparsely populated communities, the solo practitioner must cover a broad area of complaints, but also recognize when it is necessary to seek appropriate help from outside the immediate area.

HOW TO FIND THE RIGHT DOCTOR

Let us assume that you are newly arrived in town and wish to find a new physician to provide your future medical care. Prior to your departure from your previous residence, ask your current physician to recommend someone at your new location. He or she may personally know of some excellent physicians, or can find the names of qualified individuals in the *Directory of Medical Specialists* (which, incidentally, includes listings of family practice physicians). Referring physicians often supply at least three names just in case one has left the area, is retired, or is no longer accepting new patients.

The *Directory*, published every year or two, provides a geographic breakdown by city and state of each specific type of specialist. The *Directory* is often available at major public libraries and in the offices of the local county medical society. The libraries of medical schools or large hospitals are other options. If you lack immediate access to one of these libraries, call your local medical society or hospital and ask for the names of three or four specialists or generalists, depending upon your preference.

You might find it more rewarding, however, to peruse the *Directory* personally for names in your area. For each physician there is a listing of the date and place of birth, the school attended, and the hospitals at which he or she trained. Also listed are teaching positions, memberships in prestigious societies, and current hospital appointments, all of which contribute to a picture of the physician's stature in the medical community.

Board Eligibility and Certification

Not too many years ago there were still some states in which an individual could graduate from medical school and immediately obtain a license to hang up a shingle and practice just about any kind of medicine or surgery. Gradually, regulations were instituted that required at least a year's internship before a physician could practice independently. In some hospitals a two-year period of such postgraduate training was provided.

As modern medical practice became more complex, the specialties and later the subspecialties came into being. Boards of senior physicians in each specialty began to establish a set of training criteria that physicians must meet before they could be approved to practice in certain specialized branches of medicine. Today, following graduation from medical school, a physician must follow a period of prescribed training that ranges from three to as many as nine years or more for some of these specialties and subspecialties. Following the completion of training at an approved teaching hospital, the physician is then deemed "board eligible," which means he or she is eligible to take an examination, written or oral or both, in the specialty. Successful completion of the examination results in certification by that board, and the title "Diplomate" (board-certified) is conferred. (Only board-certified specialists are listed in the *Directory of Medical Specialists.*)

Patients attempting to evaluate the qualifications of a physician should be aware that many boards are now requiring periodic recertification by examination to ensure that previously certified specialists keep abreast of developments in their field in the years following their initial certification. For example, the American Board of Internal Medicine now requires that every 10 years a diplomate be reexamined to maintain his or her board certification. Other specialty boards have taken similar steps, or are about to do so.

Patients should also be aware that the term "board-eligible" can be abused. The term arose to designate the physicians who had completed their formal preparation in training and were in the process of taking the examination for certification. However, some physicians who failed the certifying examinations one or several times have continued to represent themselves as "board-eligible" for many years following their unsuccessful attempts at certification. To prevent such misrepresentation from confusing the unwary patient, many boards are beginning to impose time limits on how long this designation can be used before physicians must either obtain certification or abandon representing themselves as specialists in that field.

Hospital administrations are also taking steps to ensure that their physicians remain current in their medical knowledge. Each year, members of hospital staffs must attend a certain number of educational lectures or conferences on-site or at state or national meetings. A requisite number of credit hours must be accumulated and documented to keep these doctors in good standing on the staff.

In addition to restricting practice in certain types of specialties to those who are board-certified, some hospitals add their own requirements before allowing new members of their staffs to perform certain diagnostic or therapeutic procedures.

Following the M.D. after a physician's name, you may see the initials F.A.C.S. or F.A.C.P. The *F* stands for "fellow," and the other letters signify fellowship in the American College of Surgeons or the American College of Physicians. (The British have their royal counterparts—F.R.C.S., F.R.C.P., and so forth—and occasionally among British-trained physicians now residing in the United States such titles may be included in their listing.) The colleges were set up primarily for postgraduate education in the different specialties, although they get involved in a number of political and social issues as well. They are the major sponsors of annual conventions and many ongoing teaching programs to keep the profession abreast of developments in their field. Certification in the specialty is usually but not invariably a major requirement for fellowship.

Certification of your physician gives you some assurance that the man or woman in whose hands you are putting your health, welfare, and even life has convinced established experts in the field that he or she is possessed of adequate knowledge to practice it intelligently. It does *not* guarantee that this individual is agreeable and compassionate or even as scrupulous as you would like; all you know is that he or she has the knowledge necessary to do the job.

There certainly are good doctors who are not board-certified, but they are becoming exceedingly rare as older physicians, well established at the time the boards were initiated, either retire or die. Many of them—perhaps rightfully so—did not feel at the time that they had to prove themselves to anyone. But in the current medical climate, restrictions upon medical specialty practice are so rigid that essentially all physicians now seek board certification upon completing their training.

In the selection of your personal physician there is one other option open to you: the recommendations of friends. Bear in mind that the recommendation of a layperson does not guarantee the professional knowledge and skill of the physician. For this reason, follow up a friend's recommendation with your own investigations, as outlined previously.

Having decided upon the type of physician you want, in what framework of medical practice will you feel most comfortable? From whom will you receive the best possible care that is also the most economically favorable to you?

Solo vs. Group Practice

Physicians used to think of themselves as one of the last bastions of individuality in American life; some still do. These are likely to be solo practitioners—GPs, internists, or whatever—who are most comfortable being totally in charge of their practices, with no external interference. Today many physicians are opting instead for group practice, which allows them more leisure time as well as permitting them to share responsibility for their practice.

From your point of view, such consuming dedication as the solo practitioner usually displays may be desirable and comforting. However, aside from the obvious difficulty in finding such care these days, you have to realize that if anything should happen to your doctor, you would have to start the search for another physican, perhaps at the worst possible time.

Another negative aspect of such care is that the solo practitioner is less likely to have the benefit of consultation, formal and otherwise, that is part and parcel of group practice. For these and other reasons, usually economic, group practices have become highly popular among the medical community.

Such group practices may encompass a single specialty, such as pediatrics or orthopedic surgery, or a wide range of specialties that provide broad coverage for all the common problems, and some of the less common ones, presented by patients. A group may consist of only two or three physicians, or as many as forty to fifty, with their own office building, laboratories, and other facilities. From the patient's point of view, what a group practice may lack in exclusively personal attention may be counterbalanced by more consistent coverage and a broader range of skills available to diagnose and treat his illness.

Health Maintenance Organizations (HMOs)

Because of concerns about rising medical costs under the fee-for-service system, prepaid health care under Health Maintenance Organizations (HMOs) has been encouraged by the federal government, some insurers, and others responsible for meeting the health-care costs of the public. Under this system, you or your employer pays a fixed fee to an HMO each year, and for that fee the plan provides you with whatever health care you need. HMOs are one of the most rapidly growing segments of the health-care industry in recent years.

Advantages. The first three advantages of HMO membership could be stated as cost, cost, and then cost. Under such a plan you are reasonably assured that, whatever happens in the year ahead, you and your insurance company will not suddenly be deluged with bills.

In the fee-for-service system, the more services doctors supply, the more they receive in payment. So there is an incentive for the doctor to perform whatever test or procedure might be useful in diagnosing or treating your problem.

Under the HMO system, the whole idea is to contain costs, and therefore unnecessary laboratory work and hospitalizations are scrupulously avoided. However, for any diagnostic work that must be done, HMO physicians concerned about the cost factor for their patients don't have to worry that they may be adding to their patients' financial burdens.

Disadvantages. The main disadvantage of HMOs is that your choice of physicians is limited to those within the plan. Physician salaries in HMOs are usually lower than those in the fee-for-service area. This may keep out some highly skilled specialists who would be in high demand under either system. To counter this, some HMOs allow physicians on their panels who maintain separate practices that are run on a fee-for-service basis. Unfortunately, such physicians may be temped to give more time and attention to patients in their fee-for-service practices than to those in the prepaid HMO. In any case, you will have to pay the customary fee-for-service payment to any specialist you use who is not enrolled in the HMO.

Avoiding unnecessary lab work or hospitalization is frequently an advantage of the HMO system, but the other side of the coin is that, to save money, HMOs may apply so much pressure to limit diagnostic services that even necessary diagnostic work is not done. Some HMO physicians (usually *ex*-HMO physicians) have complained that pay disincentives as well as other pressures to hold down costs restricted their ability to practice in what they thought was an adequately responsible manner. Finally, restrictions on reimbursements allowed by government insurers (Medicare, Medicaid) for various types of medical care have caused losses to many HMOs, forcing them to restrict or cancel coverage for certain types of patients.

The final story on HMOs and their role in American medicine is not yet in. In future years, regulatory action in the interests of the consumer may control them better. Right now there may be significant differences between various plans that are open to you. Evaluate each one carefully before enrolling—ask questions, and do some comparison shopping.

HEALTH CARE INSURANCE

The increasing costs of medical care become very real when you suddenly have to bear them personally. In a country with a population of around 250 million, all but approximately 37 million Americans have some kind of health insurance. Very few, however, know just how good that coverage is until they are hospitalized for a major illness and the bills begin to arrive. Most physicians are scarcely more knowledgeable about this than are their patients. Even for such common coverages as "the blues"—Blue Shield for the doctor's services, Blue Cross for the hospital and laboratory bills—and Medicare and Medicaid, there are sufficient variations to confuse anyone who does not deal with them almost on a full-time basis. But the following list of suggestions may prove helpful.

1. Individual coverage always costs much more than do group plans. If you are a member of *any* group (veterans, union, fraternal organizations, etc.) don't overlook the possibility that it might have a group plan under which you and your family can be covered.

2. Although it may not be easy to understand all aspects of your health policy, you should be able to determine what physician fees and hospital services are included and what the deductibles are for such categories. For example, if you are considering any elective medical treatment, arrange to have it done within the calendar year in which you have already met the deductible amount required under your policy.

3. If you are retiring or leaving an organization under which you enjoyed a good health plan, you may be allowed to continue as a member even after your departure. The federal Consolidated Omnibus Reconciliation Act of 1985 (COBRA) contains provisions for extension of such benefits at the group rate for variable periods following your separation. Under this same act,

an employer has a responsibility to provide the divorced spouse of an employee with group insurance for certain periods of time following the divorce.

4. Your basic health insurance undoubtedly will have limitations in the number of hospital days allowed in one year, in the types of medical/surgical coverage, and so forth. Major medical coverage, usually purchased at rates lower than basic coverage, picks up where your basic coverage leaves off. With increasing restrictions now being placed on basic coverage by financially strapped third-party payers, major medical coverage is probably an essential part of anyone's personal or family health insurance plan.

5. Don't be intimidated by the deluge of bills you may receive after a hospitalization. Hospital bills and doctor bills will be submitted to you separately; so will the bills for certain services—X rays, for example. The same will apply to procedures involving your cardiologist or surgeon. Moreover, you will see the names of doctors you never knew existed—usually radiologists, pathologists, or others who have been genuinely involved in your care. Nevertheless, you should check all the bills you receive and make inquiries if you feel the need.

6. Keep good records of all your bills. When you submit them to an insurance company to process the claim, be sure to keep a photocopy of each bill for your own records, just in case the insurance company has no record of ever having received the first bill.

7. Do not overlook the fact that although you might not be covered for a certain service under your own plan, your spouse's superior plan may include the coverage. Furthermore, when your own plan allows for only partial payment, your wife's plan may allow for payment of the balance. This is another reason to keep copies of bills as well as correspondence from various insurers and billing agencies.

8. Often there is a person in your doctor's office who is an expert on medical insurance and focuses on this aspect of the practice. Don't hesitate to consult with that person if you have any difficulties.

9. One way to check on the adequacy of your coverage is to ask a coworker or a friend who is under the same plan, and

who has been recently hospitalized, if the plan lived up to expectations. You may learn about gaps in the coverage and take steps to counter the problem in advance.

10. If you have a chronic illness that is covered under your current plan, you may not be able to include coverage for it under a new plan. In such instances it may be to your advantage to make every effort to hold on to your present coverage, even if it involves conversion to single coverage rather than a group plan under your present company.

11. If you switch health-insurance plans, there may be a prolonged waiting period before coverage under the new plan takes effect, perhaps many months. In particular, coverage for pregnancies often includes this type of delay.

12. Don't let the insurance companies intimidate you or wear you down. Policyholders are often discouraged from pursuing what is, after all, their rightful reimbursement. If you can, try to look upon the whole process as a challenging "game" that you can win if you persist.

SURGERY

Getting a Second Opinion

In the aftermath of a major accident, extensive surgery may be required immediately. At other times the surgery is elective; you have some time to decide whether or not you want the surgery, and, if so, who will be your surgeon.

Your first question should be, "Are there alternatives to surgery?" If there are, what are the current statistics regarding the success of these approaches? Such alternatives should be compared with the curative or merely palliative effects of surgical intervention.

Whenever the need for surgical treatment arises, there is much to be said for getting a second opinion. This option may even be required by your health-insurance plan before you undergo any elective surgery. Or it may be a completely informal undertaking on your part, in which you simply request the name of someone in the field from your primary-care physician.

This second doctor, usually a specialist, can examine you, review the laboratory data related to your illness, and then make his or her own recommendation. Do not be embarrassed to tell your doctor you want a second opinion; given the risks and expense of surgery, it is an accepted and even a recommended method of confirming a diagnosis. Make sure that all pertinent records are made freely available to the second reviewing physician, so that he or she will not need to repeat any diagnostic tests.

A word of caution about second opinions: The search for absolute certainty can be overdone. Sometimes second opinions become third and fourth opinions, with great cost to the patient in terms of time, money, and anguish for himself and his family. After all, there are times when the findings are so clear-cut and the indications for surgery so unequivocal that no responsible physician would opt for any other course—for example, in the case of a small, localized cancer that has not yet spread and for which surgery could result in a cure. At other times, by the time the question of surgery is brought up, your problem has already been reviewed by a panel of medical and surgical experts who convene periodically at hospital conferences to evaluate such problems and make recommendations. If the panel was unanimous in their decision for or against surgery, this information should be presented to you. If there was disagreement, you should be aware of both sides of the issue.

Choosing a Surgeon

Surgery has been recommended, the second opinion concurs, and you have decided to go ahead with it. How do you know you have the right surgeon? Feel free, when you meet with the surgeon, to ask about how many such operations of this type he or she has performed. What has been the mortality rate? What complications are possible, and what are their frequencies? Is the surgery completely curative, or is there a chance that even with surgery the problem may recur?

Let us assume you have decided in favor of surgery and you have selected a surgeon to undertake it. There is still one question unaddressed: the fee.

Major surgery can run into many thousands of dollars. Although insurance companies and Medicare are often rather generous in their fee assignments for such undertakings, you should always be clear beforehand about whether or not the surgeon's fee is more than the coverage. Although physicians in general are often inexpert about insurance matters, when it comes to specific major surgical procedures, the doctor in question is often fully aware of the extent of coverage, especially for the major third-party payers. To save yourself future grief, settle *in advance* with the surgeon whether or not the fee will be covered fully by insurance. If, for any reason, the surgeon feels that the assigned fee is insufficient, ascertain the amount you will be responsible for paying. If there is financial hardship, make it known to the surgeon at this time, and ask for some kind of adjustment in the fee. Most surgeons will make allowances for your financial difficulties and either offer a reduction in their rate or an extension of the time over which you can pay them.

In the Hospital

There is probably nothing more depressing in modern life than for someone in full possession of his faculties to become, quite suddenly, a hospital patient. Once you enter the doors of most hospitals, all autonomy is suddenly lost. Your sleeping and waking hours are predetermined by others; your diet is manipulated without your consent; strange people pass in and out of your room uninvited; you are picked at, poked, and pummeled in various ways. The final mortification is the removal of all civilized garments and their replacement with an unironed gown that opens in the back to expose your backside at the most inopportune times.

It doesn't help much to know that all this is being done for your benefit. It remains a very stressful and discomforting experience even under the best of circumstances.

As things are, one can only attempt to impart to the health-care profession an appreciation of this sense of humiliation on the patient's part, and to advise you on how best to cope if you are ever hospitalized.

How a Hospital Functions

Your personal doctor, no matter how dedicated, will for the most part be only a fleeting figure in the course of your hospital day. He or she will visit for a few moments in the morning or evening on hospital rounds, order the appropriate tests and medications, and, except in the case of an emergency, disappear until the next day.

It is the nurses who see that you get to the right lab at the right time, administer medications, and check your vital signs to chart your progress. It is they who will be on the phone to your doctor or others involved in your care. It is they who will be responsible for your creature comforts, especially if you are bedridden.

Because of the frequent lack of adequate nursing coverage, the ratio between nurses and patients is often suboptimal. What this means to you as a patient is that you may not be watched as closely as you should be; you may even miss medications; and you certainly won't have many of your more unofficial requests attended to.

Even when it appears that staffing is adequate, it is often less efficient than it should be. Many nurses, to gain better control of their working hours and conditions, have left the staffs of hospitals and signed up with nursing agencies. As the nursing department of a hospital foresees a shortage for a particular shift, an agency nurse will be brought in to fill the gap. This nurse has no prior knowledge of your condition and is often ignorant of just where things are on the hospital ward.

As a patient, sometimes it may help to ensure your well-being with private duty nursing, especially if you are confined to bed. Round-the-clock private nursing is extremely expensive and rarely necessary. The usual nursing shifts run from 7:00 A.M. to 3:00 P.M., from 3:00 P.M. to 11:00 P.M., and from 11:00 P.M. to 7:00 A.M. Staffing is usually best for the first shift, and you are often sleeping during the third. So it is often during the three-to-eleven shift that you are likely to suffer most from inadequate nurse staffing, and when the engagement of private duty nursing might be advisable. You could also encourage members of your family to come to the hospital and help during these hours. Under certain circumstances your doctor can order exemption from visiting-hour rules to permit this if you request it.

Interns and residents. Some hospital patients refuse to let anyone but their personal physician treat them. This attitude, in the setting of many critical illnesses, could be interpreted as an inadvertent death wish. In case a new symptom appears, or some change in your condition occurs in the middle of the night, it will not be your private doctor called to the bedside first, but rather an intern, resident, house physician, or even a physician's assistant (a so-called PA) who will evaluate you before contacting your physician. If the doctor or assistant has not previously examined you, he or she may be ill-prepared to judge whether the changes that have occurred are alarming or not.

Medical students are not in hospitals simply to learn from you as a patient, although that is a vital part of their training. They are also there to assist your physician in getting you well. Occasionally they may even pick up some clues to your illness that your doctor might have missed, or they may suggest a test or type of therapy that your physician may wish to pursue.

In teaching hospitals, you may experience visits from various medical consultants, depending upon the nature of your illness. They will often bring with them their own retinue of students and trainees. It may prove distressing to you to have so many different individuals poring over you, especially when you are incapacitated. However, a good general guide to care in a hospital is that the less of this type of attention you receive, the greater the likelihood that your care will be inferior. On the other hand, when you are sick and in pain, your desire for rest must be respected, and excessive visiting of this sort should and can be curtailed on orders of your personal physician.

Patients' rights. Matching the number of doctors you encounter in the hospital will be the number of forms you are asked to sign. Paramount among these are the **informed consents** required before the undertaking of certain procedures. Other than surgery, these procedures frequently involve invasive diagnostic measures such as the placing of catheters in the heart or great vessels, or diagnostic radiological procedures involving the injection of certain substances that outline anatomical structures on X-ray film. Certain potentially hazardous tests, such as exercise stress testing, require your informed consent, as does the insertion of needles or other instruments for getting tissue or fluid samples (other than simple drawing of blood from a vein or artery in the arm or leg).

There are several basic components of this agreement between patient and doctor. Informed consents include the following:

- an explanation of what is to be done, and why
- a description of possible risks
- an explanation of the benefits to be obtained
- disclosure of possible diagnostic or therapeutic alternatives
- an offer to answer any questions about the procedure
- in experimental procedures, disclosure of that fact; the patient also must be informed in such cases that he or she may withdraw at any time

In view of the magnitude of the malpractice problem, physicians today usually take great pains to clarify these issues with patients. Patients are similarly sensitive to the possibilities of their rights being abridged. Yet misunderstandings about informed consent continue to occur. A presidential commission on ethical problems in medicine has suggested that the concept of "informed consent" be replaced by one of "shared decision making," in which a collaborative effort can be made by the physician and the patient in the latter's best interests. This certainly seems a more humane approach than the legalistic "informed consent," although, in the final analysis, as one wise physician has put it, the patient's real protection is the conscience and compassion of his physician.

There are other aspects of the individual's rights that need to be respected. For one, confidentiality of information is a long-standing tradition in medicine that needs to be maintained. Patients also should not be denied the right to seek other professional opinions. Participation in any sort of research program should be made clear to the patient, along with the option to remove himself from it at any time. Access to hospital records as well as office records should be assured so that tests need not be repeated and other physicians engaged by the patient can be fully informed about past medical history. (Release forms signed by the patient for information to be sent elsewhere are legally required.)

The right to decline any treatment cannot be denied even if, in the eyes of the patient's physician, such refusal might very well result in the death of the patient. Decisions to decline treatment are especially important when further treatment can provide only questionable survival benefits and/or symptomatic relief to the patient. In advanced terminal cancer or prolonged coma, repeated efforts to resuscitate in cases of respiratory or cardiac arrest may not always be in the patient's best interest. When the patient is incapable of saying "enough," the family may instruct the attending physician to write "do not resuscitate" orders. Preferable to this, to relieve families of any potential guilt, patients may elect to prepare living wills (see page 234), making their own personal feelings about such matters known in advance to all concerned.

Length of hospitalization. Some years ago a system called Diagnostic Related Groupings (DRG) was devised for the purposes of classifying and dealing with various diseases. Later, first the state of New Jersey and then other entities (most notably Medicare in 1983) adopted the DRG system as part of an effort to reduce hospital costs by determining how many days of hospitalization on the average were required for each one of more than 500 different disorders and diseases. On the basis of these calculations, depending upon the coded diagnosis only, so many days of hospitalization would be allowed for purposes of patient reimbursement. For example, if you have "disease A," only five days may be allowed for your hospitalization; if you have "disease B," then eight hospital days; "disease C," two days, etc. For any days of hospitalization exceeding the prescribed number, there is no reimbursement to the hospital, which must then absorb the costs of the additional days spent treating the patient.

The effect of such restrictions has been to pressure hospitals to pressure doctors to discharge patients within the prescribed periods. Doctors complained from the outset that such pressure would inevitably lead to their patients being discharged both "quicker and sicker." In attempts to address such objections, modifications of the program have been instituted. Still, reports of potential harm to patients have appeared in the medical literature. The full story is not in, but given the widespread nature of DRG as a basis for hospital reimbursement in the United States today, every medical consumer should be aware that such concerns may affect one of his own future hospitalizations.

ALTERNATIVE MEDICINE

So far we have considered only orthodox, main-line **allopathic medicine** as it is generally practiced in the United States today. What have come to be called "alternative" approaches to health care have achieved some popularity among certain segments of the American public. Some of these practices are more acceptable than others; some are downright fraudulent and should be avoided at all costs.

Osteopathy

Originally based on principles involving bone-setting, magnetism, and certain other unconventional approaches to the treatment of disease, osteopathy has gradually incorporated more conventional methods of diagnosis and treatment into its practice, while eliminating the more unusual practices that once characterized it. Although many early osteopaths were not even physicians, osteopathic schools now number 15 within the United States, and incorporate most of the normal medical curriculum in the training of their students. In some instances osteopathic physicians will even take their first two years of basic science training with regular (allopathic) medical students before completing their clinical years at osteopathic hospitals.

Because of such developments, there has been a trend to incorporate Doctors of Osteopathy (D.O.'s) into mainstream medicine. In 1962 in California, for instance, graduates of osteopathic schools were, for the first time, awarded M.D. degrees. The American Medical Association has for years been in favor of this trend. There has been some resistance to this, however, on the part of those osteopaths who believe they represent a distinctive type of primary-care physician whose separate identity they wish to maintain. They feel that emphasis on the body's natural ability to defend itself, along with the osteopath's ability to apply manipulative skills in the treatment of many common musculoskeletal problems, offers an important ingredient in the field of family practice other than that provided by allopathic medical practitioners.

From the patient's standpoint, the care of an osteopath may be preferable to that of the ordinary GP or internist, especially if recurrent musculoskeletal problems, successfully handled by that osteopath, constitute a major feature of his health care.

There is a potential downside to osteopathic care. Specialty types of care have not developed among osteopaths anywhere to the degree they have among the main body of physicians, who often staff the university hospitals associated with medical schools. Osteopaths frequently run their own hospitals. In the latter setting, highly skilled specialty care is less likely to be available to you.

Acupuncture

Acupuncture today is looked upon as more of a minor adjunct to medical care than a separate form of therapy, as it is traditionally viewed in China. Although poorly understood in the West, acupuncture techniques are used by some generalists, anethesiologists, and others for the relief of pain in multiple conditions. (In China it has also been used as the primary form of pain control even in major abdominal and thoracic surgery.) In the United States and Great Britain, physicians often utilize electrode stimulation rather than the traditional needles inserted at the prescribed control points on the body.

Holistic Medicine

In response to growing dissatisfaction with the restrictive and impersonal approach to patient care that has characterized much of modern scientific medicine, an emerging group of physicians have championed a more humanistic type of practice. Representing more of an attitude than a separate system of health care, holistic medicine emphasizes, in addition to the scientific application of medical knowledge, factors such as emotional health, diet, exercise, good personal habits, and the psychological aspects of illness. The central idea is that we should treat the whole patient, not the illness.

Such efforts are laudable to the extent that delivery of good medical care improves the collaboration between patient and doctor. In the hands of some proponents, this approach becomes more "holy" than "whole," however, and in such cases it tends to engender some skepticism on the part of other medical observers.

QUESTIONABLE APPROACHES TO HEALTH CARE

Whatever the scientific achievements of modern medicine, the failure to communicate these adequately to the public has allowed certain medical and nonmedical individuals of questionable skill and motivation to continue to attract patients to their doors. The offerings of such practitioners take on special appeal when modern medicine fails to meet the patient's expectations, or where the patient has reached a terminal state of his disease and conventional medicine can no longer offer any hope for an ultimate cure.

Chiropractors

There is perhaps no opinion more difficult for the physician to render than an opinion on chiropractors that all might consider fair and equable. Medical doctors were all raised professionally to look upon chiropractors as quacks at best, and the internal squabbling among different chiropractic factions has not made a fair judgment any easier. The "straights" among them have adhered narrowly to the practice of spinal adjustments and manipulations. The "mixers" include physical therapy—heat, water, massage, and some herbal remedies and/or dietary prescriptions.

However contentious they have been among themselves, chiropractors have proved undeniably resourceful as a group in the courts, cowing the opposition of organized medicine into silence. They have also succeeded politically and economically, having been granted reimbursement for services by Medicare in 1972 despite an adverse recommendation from the Surgeon General.

Unlike other types of healers, such as homeopaths and osteopaths, chiropractors are unlikely ever to become absorbed into the mainstream of medicine. This is because the majority continue to abjure drug treatment of disease at a time when it represents a major bastion of conventional medical therapy.

Yet it is undeniable that chiropractors enjoy success among a variety of patients, many of whom are intelligent, well educated, and certainly capable of affording conventional medical care. How can one account for this? Obviously patients are getting results from their chiropractors that they cannot or have not received from conventional practitioners. The reasons for this are probably multiple and include the self-limiting nature of some of their complaints and the personal care and attention that patients may find at the chiropractor's office and not at the M.D.'s. Furthermore, in addition to spinal manipulation, chiropractors administer heat or prescribe exercise and other accepted modalities of treatment that may, in themselves, be effective in many pain syndromes.

What is most troubling to the medical profession is the limited extent of their training. Requirements to enter schools of chiropractic are much less stringent than those for medical school. Only recently have some schools of chiropractic required even a bachelor's degree for admission.

There are reports in the medical literature about severe permanent paralysis in patients who have undergone chiropractic manipulations, but given the large numbers of these performed on a daily basis, such mishaps are probably quite rare. Of greater concern is the potential delay in the diagnosis and proper treatment of many diseases for which good medical therapy *is* available. Many physicians fear that, unlike osteopaths (with whom they are sometimes confused by the laity), most chiropractors are unlikely to recognize many of these illnesses when they encounter them. Perhaps such fears are unjustified, since many patients seek the help of the chiropractor only after the medical profession has failed to relieve the lower back pain and other musculoskeletal problems for which chiropractors are most commonly patronized by their patients.

Finally, patients recognize that many effective drugs are now available that may be useful in treating their complaints. As long as chiropractors refuse to prescribe them, the patient will seek the appropriate source of such medication.

Homeopathy

Although much less popular now than in the past, homeopathy is based on the principle that disease may be treated by administration of extremely minute doses of substances that would, in healthy persons, produce the same ill effects when given in large doses (for example, a small amount of laxative to treat diarrhea). In earlier times, when many of our medications did more harm than good, homeopathy was probably preferable to many of the conventional medical treatments of the day. With the introduction of effective modern medicines, it has fallen out of favor generally.

Spiritual Healing

There is no doubt that personal factors—spiritual ones, if you will—seem to influence the outcome of illnesses. There do indeed seem to be some patients with such a will to live that it appears to affect the outcome of their illness in a positive way, and others who simply seem to give up the fight. The power of supernatural healing, however, is less convincing. To put it bluntly, when it comes to a pneumococcal pneumonia, for example, the power of prayer is no match for a few good doses of penicillin. Still, a case can be made that a positive outlook, a cheery disposition, and ridding oneself of such negative emotions as anger and guilt can contribute to your good health and recovery.

AVOIDING HEALTH QUACKERY

The advance of medicine in recent decades has been truly remarkable. In the postwar half of the century, drugs for the treatment of hypertension and cancer, as well as a variety of new surgical techniques, have completely transformed the practice of medicine.

And yet, with all our new learning comes realization about the immense gaps in our knowledge. When two apparently quite similar patients come down with a disease and are given the same treatment, why does one recover and the other succumb? When a certain disease begins to spread in epidemic proportions, why do some people contract it and others, equally exposed, escape it completely? Why do certain diseases, such as stomach cancer, gradually decrease in incidence and other new ones, such as AIDS, spring forth almost out of nowhere? Perhaps it is for reasons such as these, in part, that quackery continues to flourish, especially in instances in which conventional medical treatment has failed.

Among terminal cancer patients especially, nostrums such as Krebiozen and Laetrile eventually proved completely worthless, and have had their day. Currently, AIDS patients, with no cure in sight, are prone to victimization as well.

How is one to avoid potential medical quackery? There are some danger markers that are typical of such practices and deserve attention from the health-care consumer:

1. Any treatment that must be given *only* in the home or office of some doctor or other professed healer, rather than in a hospital setting, should alert you to potential fraud. Hospital committees are very circumspect before allowing the introduction of new drugs. Surgical or other procedures also undergo meticulous scrutiny. These are protections you should not forgo.

2. Be especially cautious if the one administering your medical procedure complains that organized medicine is against the treatment because those doctors are only interested in protecting their own interests.

3. If a new "miracle worker" cannot refer you to any published studies demonstrating the efficacy of his or her treatment, it may be a hoax.

4. Check for the certification or hospital staff privileges of the practitioner in whose hands you are placing your welfare. If he or she does not meet the usual criteria of acceptability, there is usually a good reason why.

MEDICAL MALPRACTICE

In addition to those quacks who are guilty of deliberate misrepresentation, there are well-meaning incompetents in the medical community who may do you more harm than good. One study estimated the number to be about 5 percent of the total.

Part of the problem is that even after being exposed as incompetent, some doctors manage to go on providing inferior medical care. The medical profession does not have a police force to travel around the country, making sure that such a physician does not go to another state and set up a practice. A call to your local medical society will either confirm that the doctor you are seeing is duly licensed, or they can set in motion the legal steps necessary to close him or her down.

Recently there has been a new development for the protection of the public against medical malfeasance. As of the summer of 1989, a data bank has collected information on all malpractice judgments and disciplinary actions, and has made it available to all hospitals considering the applications of newly arrived physicians. All hospitals will be required to check on new staff applicants in this way. Lawyers representing malpractice claimants will also have access to this information.

Most patients, according to many surveys, express satisfaction with their own doctors, and continue to hold the profession in generally high esteem despite misgivings about "bad apples" and other negative aspects of medical care. Nevertheless, malpractice insurance coverage in some medical specialties has exceeded $100,000 annually in some areas, and behind every such suit, justified or not, lurks the threat of a ruined career. It is important to recognize that the enormous costs of malpractice litigation are ultimately borne by patients as a group.

Though no instance of actual malpractice should go unpunished, it is in the interests of patients as well as physicians that unjustified suits be eliminated as much as possible. They are costly for insurance companies to defend, and often result in nuisance-value settlements that have no basis in fairness. It must be recognized that the failure of a particular treatment is in itself not evidence of malpractice. To insist otherwise is to paralyze medicine and drive from it all but the most insensitive and unimaginative drones, those willing to withhold all treatment that promises less than a 100-percent chance of success.

Index